UPDATE ON HEARING LOSS

Edited by **Fayez Bahmad Jr.**

Update On Hearing Loss

http://dx.doi.org/10.5772/59528
Edited by Fayez Bahmad Jr.

Contributors

Sidheshwar Pandey, Mukeshwar Pandey, Miguel Hyppolito, Eduardo Massuda, Ana Cristina Coelho, Alcione Brasolotto, Daniela Medved, Stavros Hatzopoulos, Henryk Skarzynski, Piotr H Skarzynski, Frank Richter, Edeltraut Emmerich, Marcus Engelmann, Melanie Rohmann, Miriam Furst, Waleed Alshuaib, Jasim Al-Kandari, Sonia Hasan, Klára Procházková, Aleš Hahn, Ivan Šejna, Petr Schalek, Jozef Rosina, Luiz Alberto Alves Mota, Paula Leitão, Paulo Barros, Ana Maria Dos Anjos Carneiro-Leão, Larissa Vilela

Published by InTech

Janeza Trdine 9, 51000 Rijeka, Croatia

Publishing Process Manager Iva Lipovic

Technical Editor InTech DTP team

Cover InTech Design team

First published December, 2015

Printed in Croatia

Additional hard copies can be obtained from orders@intechopen.com

Update On Hearing Loss, Edited by Fayez Bahmad Jr.

p. cm.

ISBN 978-953-51-2195-4

For EU product safety concerns:
IN TECH d.o.o., Prolaz Marije Krucifikse Kozulić 3, 51000 Rijeka, Croatia,
info@intechopen.com or visit our website at intechopen.com.

Meet the editor

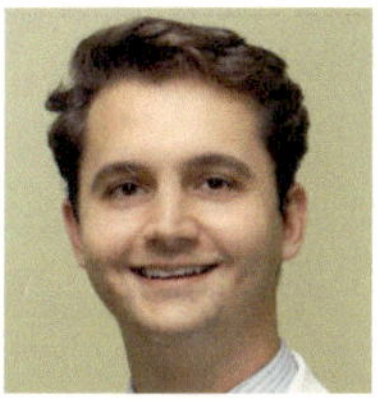

Professor Dr. Fayez Bahmad Jr. is the Editor in Chief of *The International Tinnitus Journal*. He completed the ENT Residency Program at the University of Brasilia Hospital (Otolaryngology) and received his PhD at the University of Brasilia Medical School under the orientation of Prof. Carlos A. Oliveira, MD, PhD. Professor Oliveira is well known for establishing one of the most successful research groups in Otology in Brazil and South America. Professor Dr. Fayez Bahmad Jr. was awarded the prestigious Schuknecht Prize at The International Otopathology Society Meeting held in Boston in 2003. He was a Fellow in Otology and Neurotology at the Massachusetts Eye and Ear Infirmary and Fellow in Human Genetics at Seidman Laboratory, Department of Genetics, both at Harvard Medical School when he was engaged in projects under the mentorship of Prof. Saumil N. Merchant, MD, PhD, one of the foremost professors and researchers in otology and otopathology in the Harvard Medical School.

Contents

Preface

Update on Hearing Loss is directed toward medical students, clinicians, and otolaryngologists and provides detailed information on hearing loss, many different forms of hearing loss, and their treatment as well as an overview of what is new and known about their pathophysiology.

Accordingly, this book does not cover all the different theories and management strategies of hearing loss, but it does present up-to-date information for those who deal with hearing loss in their clinical practice, such as otolaryngologists, neurologists, psychiatrists, neurosurgeons, clinical audiologists, dentists, and psychologists.

This book encompasses both the theoretical background of the different forms of hearing loss and detailed knowledge on state-of-the-art treatment, written for clinicians by specialists and researchers. Realizing the complexity of hearing loss has highlighted the importance of interdisciplinary research. Therefore, all the authors contributing to *Update on Hearing Loss* were chosen from many different specialties of medicine, like surgery, psychology, and neuroscience, and came from diverse areas of expertise, such as neurology, neurosurgery, audiology and speech therapy, otolaryngology, psychiatry, clinical and experimental psychology, pharmacology, dentistry, and neuroscience.

Many structures of the body, such as the ear, the auditory nervous system, the somatosensory system, other parts of the brain, and muscles of the head and the neck, are directly or indirectly involved in different forms of hearing loss. Treating and understanding the pathology of hearing loss require better knowledge of otopathology and the involvement of many specialties of medicine, such as surgery, psychology, and neuroscience.

Hearing loss may occur due to genetic defects, presbycusis, viral or bacterial infection, temporal bone trauma, noise exposure, or administration of ototoxical agents. Hearing loss is often accompanied by symptoms such as hyperacusis (lowered tolerance to sound) and distortion of sounds. Affective disorders such as phonophobia (fear of sound) and depression often occur in individuals with severe hearing loss.

Chapter 1 provides the reader with current knowledge on the Cochlear Model for Hearing Loss.

Chapter 2 describes the newest Classification of Hearing Loss.

Chapter 3 is an Update on Etiology and Epidemiology of Hearing Loss.

Chapter 4 discusses the Advances in Genetic Diagnosis and Treatment of Hearing Loss.

Chapter 5 is about Hearing Loss in Infectious and Contagious Diseases.

Chapter 6 presents a critical overview of Hearing Loss and Its Impact on Voice.

Chapter 7 discusses the components of Noise-Induced Hearing Loss.

Chapter 8 offers new alternative treatments of Tinnitus as Therapy with Laser and EGb 761.

Chapter 9 presents the Technological Advances in Universal Neonatal Hearing Screening.

Chapter 10 describes Cochlear Implantation on Hearing-Impaired Patients.

It is a huge challenge to translate the results from basic research into clinical practice, and all the authors have attempted to present the pathophysiological model in a clear way. Still, the principles on which it is based and its mechanisms are complex, and their understanding requires knowledge from various areas of neuroscience; the fact that hearing loss is not a simple disease necessitates the involvement of several disciplines of health care.

The editor would like to thank Ms. Iva Lipović for her support in the preparation of this book.

Special thanks go to the chapter authors.

Fayez Bahmad Jr., MD, PhD
President of the Brasiliense Institute of Otolaryngology
Professor at the Health Science Faculty,
University of Brasilia,
Brasil

Section 1

Basis of Hearing Loss

Chapter 1

Cochlear Model for Hearing Loss

Miriam Furst

Additional information is available at the end of the chapter

http://dx.doi.org/10.5772/61189

Abstract

In many psychoacoustical tasks, hearing-impaired subjects display abnormal audiograms and poor understanding of speech compared to normal listeners. Existing models that explain the performance of the hearing impaired indicate that possible sources for cochlear hearing loss may be the dysfunction of the outer and inner hair cells. In this study, a model of the auditory system is introduced. It includes two stages: (1) a nonlinear time domain cochlear model with active outer hair cells that are driven by the tectorial membrane motion and (2) a synaptic model that generates the auditory nerve instantaneous rate as a response to the basilar membrane motion and is affected by the inner hair cell transduction efficiency. The model can fit both a normal auditory system and an abnormal auditory system with easily induced pathologies.

In typical psychoacoustical detection experiments, the ability of subjects to perceive a minimum difference in a physical property is measured. We use the model presented here to predict these performances by assuming that the brain behaves as an optimal processor that estimates a particular physical parameter. The performance of the optimal processor is derived by calculating its lower bound. Since neural activity is described as a nonhomogeneous Poisson process whose instantaneous rate was derived, the Cramer–Rao lower bound can be analytically obtained for both rate coding and all information coding.

We compared the model predictions of normal and abnormal cochleae to human thresholds of pure tones in quiet and in the presence of background noise.

Keywords: Cochlear model, outer hair cell, audiogram, hearing impairment, auditory nerve

1. Introduction

When sound waves enter the ear, they cause the basilar membrane (BM) that is located in the inner ear to vibrate. Since each place on the BM is tuned to a specific characteristic frequency

(CF), the BM is able to separate the frequency components of sounds. The BM vibrations excite both the outer hair cells (OHC) and the inner hair cells (IHC). The OHCs act as local amplifiers, while the IHCs transduce the sound-induced vibrations into electrical impulses that propagate up the auditory cortex through the fiber tracks of the auditory pathway where the neural information is processed in a set of nuclei located in the auditory brainstem.

Damage can occur to the auditory system at any point along the auditory pathway. One of the most common impairments is OHC loss, frequently due to noise exposure. Often, when there is OHC loss , it is followed by IHC loss. Various diseases or old age can also injure different neurons along the auditory pathway.

Hearing impairment is characterized by abnormal audiograms and poor understanding of speech. The most frequent complaint is the inability to understand speech in a noisy environment. In many psychoacoustical tasks, hearing-impaired subjects yield lower thresholds than normal listeners (review by Moore [1]). For example, in monaural experiments, hearing-impaired subjects perform poorly in frequency discrimination tasks and in signal detection with a noisy background.

Models explaining the performance of hearing-impaired people [e.g., 2–9] indicate that the possible sources for cochlear hearing loss are the dysfunction of the outer hair cells and the loss of inner hair cells. The dysfunction of the OHCs reduces the gain of the active mechanism, which then tends to broaden the tuning curve and decrease the nonlinear effects. However, these models do not adequately predict hearing impairment performance [10, 11].

The purpose of this chapter is to introduce a comprehensive, nonlinear time domain cochlear model [6, 12–14], followed by a model of the auditory nerve (AN) response [7, 13, 16, 17] that can be used to predict hearing abilities of people with normal cochlea as well as with abnormal cochlea that suffers from either OHC loss and/or IHC loss.

Quantitative psychoacoustical measures that determine the human ability to detect the smallest difference in the physical property of a stimulus are usually implemented by forced-choice experiments. This difference is referred to as a "just-noticeable difference" (JND). Siebert [18] showed that if one assumes that the brain is behaving as an optimal processor, then psychoacoustical JND measurements can be predicted from auditory nerve instantaneous rates. In this chapter, we use this approach to compare the model predictions to human hearing thresholds, both normal and impaired, in both a quiet environment and in the presence of background noise.

2. The human ear model

The mammalian ear is composed of the outer ear, the middle ear, and the inner ear. The outer ear includes the pinna, the ear canal, and the ear drum. The middle ear is an air-filled cavity behind the ear drum, which includes three small ear bones, the ossicles. The inner ear includes a snail-shaped structure, the cochlea (see schematic description in Figure 1A).The sound is directed by the outer ear through the ear canal to the eardrum. When sound strikes the ear drum, the movement is transferred through the three bones of the middle ear to a flexible tissue called the oval window, finally reaching the upper fluid-filled ducts of the cochlea (see Figure 1). The upper cochlear ducts are called scala vestibuli, and the bottom duct is referred to as scala tympani. The space between the top and bottom ducts is labeled as scala media.

The middle ear's task is to match the impedance of the sound pressure in the air to that of the fluid. Movement of the fluid inside the upper cochlear duct results in a pressure difference between the upper and lower ducts. This pressure difference in turn causes the basilar membrane (the membrane that separates the scala tympani and scala media) to move.

Two types of auditory receptor cells inhabit the scala media, the inner and outer hair cells. The defining feature of those cells is the hair bundle on top of each cell. The hair bundle comprises dozens to hundreds of streocilia, which are cylindrical actin-filled rods. The streocilia are immersed in endolymph, a fluid that is rich in potassium and characterized by an endocochlear potential of +80 mV. The streocilia move with the basilar membrane displacement. Their deflection opens mechanically gated ion channels that allow any small, positively charged ions (primarily potassium and calcium) to enter the cell. The influx of positive ions from the endolymph in the scala media depolarizes the cell, resulting in a receptor potential. The roles of the OHCs and IHCs on the function of the cochlea are very different. While the OHCs act as local amplifiers, the IHCs innervate the auditory nerve. The OHCs lay on the basilar membrane, and their upper part is embedded in a gel-like membrane, the tectorial membrane (TM). An increase in the OHC receptor potential causes a decrease in its length [19], which in turn enhances the BM movement. The hair bundles of the IHC move freely in the scala media. The change in their receptor potential opens voltage-gated calcium channels that release neurotransmitters at the basal end of the cell, which trigger action potentials in the attached nerve.

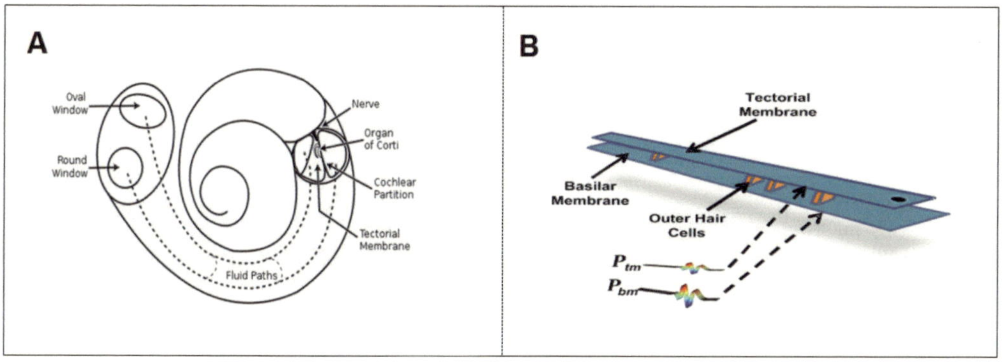

Figure 1. Schematic representation of the cochlea: (A) the snail-shaped structure of the cochlea; (B) schematic description of the Organ of Corti, emphasizing that the BM and the TM are attached by the OHCs.

Modeling the human ear requires a detailed model of the cochlea and the middle and outer ears. A common approach is to model the inner ear as a one-dimensional structure [e.g., 6, 14,

20–23] with the cochlea regarded as an uncoiled structure with two fluid-filled compartments with rigid walls that are separated by an elastic partition, the basilar membrane. The cochlear partition, whose mechanical properties are describable in terms of point-wise mass density, stiffness, and damping, is regarded as a flexible boundary between scala tympani and scala vestibuli. Thus, at every point along the cochlear duct, the pressure difference $P(x, t)$ across the partition drives the partition's velocity. By applying fundamental physical principles, such as the conservation of mass and the dynamics of deformable bodies, the differential equation for P is obtained by [e.g. 6]

$$\frac{\partial^2 P(x,t)}{\partial x^2} = \frac{2\rho\beta}{A}\frac{\partial^2 \xi_{\mathrm{bm}}(x,t)}{\partial t^2}, \tag{1}$$

where ξ_{bm} is the BM displacement, A represents the cross-sectional area of scala tympani and scala vestibuli, β is the BM width, and ρ is the density of the fluid in both the scala vestibuli and the scala tympani. The pressure on the BM (P_{bm}) is a result of both the difference in fluid pressure and the pressure caused by the OHCs (P_{ohc}). The relation between the pressures of BM, TM, and OHC is shown in Figure 1 [13], which can be interpreted as

$$\left.\begin{aligned} P_{\mathrm{bm}}(x,t) &= P(x,t) + P_{\mathrm{ohc}}(x,t) \\ 0 &= P_{\mathrm{ohc}}(x,t) + P_{\mathrm{tm}}(x,t) \end{aligned}\right\}. \tag{2}$$

The mechanical properties of both BM and TM are simulated as second-order oscillators that yield

$$\left.\begin{aligned} P_{\mathrm{bm}}(x,t) &= M_{\mathrm{bm}}(x)\cdot\frac{\partial^2\xi_{\mathrm{bm}}}{\partial t^2}(x,t) + R_{\mathrm{bm}}(x)\cdot\frac{\partial\xi_{\mathrm{bm}}}{\partial t}(x,t) + K_{\mathrm{bm}}(x)\cdot\xi_{\mathrm{bm}}(x,t) \\ P_{\mathrm{tm}}(x,t) &= M_{\mathrm{tm}}(x)\cdot\frac{\partial^2\xi_{\mathrm{tm}}}{\partial t^2}(x,t) + R_{\mathrm{tm}}(x)\cdot\frac{\partial\xi_{\mathrm{tm}}}{\partial t}(x,t) + K_{\mathrm{tm}}(x)\cdot\xi_{\mathrm{tm}}(x,t) \end{aligned}\right\}, \tag{3}$$

where K_{bm}, K_{tm}, R_{bm}, R_{tm}, M_{bm}, and M_{tm} are the effective stiffness, damping, and mass per unit area of BM and TM, respectively (see Table 1). The TM displacement is defined as ξ_{tm}.

Since the OHCs lie between the two membranes, their displacement is considered as

$$\xi_{\mathrm{ohc}} = \xi_{\mathrm{tm}} - \xi_{\mathrm{bm}}. \tag{4}$$

Each OHC is modeled by two sections, the apical and basal parts. The apical part is directed toward the endolymph of the gap between the TM and the reticular lamina (RL), while the basolateral part is embedded in the perilymph next to the supporting cells that are aligned along the BM. When the OHCs' stereocilia move due to the relative displacement of the BM and the TM, the conductance of the apical part of the OHC is affected, which in turn causes a flow of potassium and calcium ions to the endolymph. Thus, a voltage drop is developed on the basal part of the OHC membrane [24].

An outer hair cell model is described by an equivalent electrical circuit in Figure 2 [6, 25]. The apical part is presented by its variable conductance ($G_a \approx \alpha \cdot \xi_{\text{ohc}}$) and its constant capacitance (C_a), while the basal part is presented by its constant conductance and capacitance, G_b and C_b, respectively. The electrical potential of the endolymph is V_{sm}=80 mV, and the perilymph resting potential is $\psi_0 = -70$ mV. Solving the equivalent electrical circuit by using Kirchhoff laws [6] yields the differential equation for ψ_{ohc}, the OHC's membrane voltage:

$$\frac{d\psi_{\text{ohc}}}{dt} + \omega_{\text{ohc}} \cdot (\psi - \psi_0) = \eta \cdot \xi_{\text{ohc}}, \tag{5}$$

where $\omega_{\text{ohc}} \approx G_b / C_b = 1000$ Hz, which represents the cutoff frequency of the OHC's membrane and $\eta = \alpha \cdot V_{\text{sm}} / (C_b + C_a) = \text{const.}$ (see Table 1).

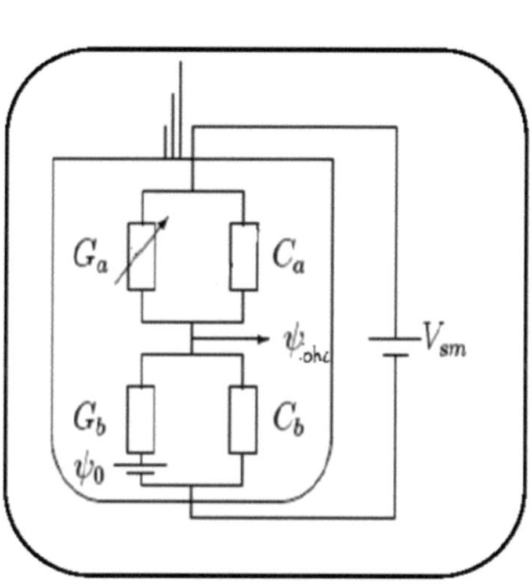

Figure 2. The equivalent electrical circuit of the outer hair cell.

An OHC's length changes due to the electrical potential developed on the OHC membrane and is defined as Δl_{ohc}. It is usually described as a sigmoid function [26–28]:

$$\Delta l_{\text{ohc}} = \alpha_s \frac{e^{(-2\cdot\alpha_l\cdot\psi)} - 1}{e^{(-2\cdot\alpha_l\cdot\psi)} + 1} = \alpha_s \tanh(-\alpha_l \cdot \psi), \tag{6}$$

where α_l and α_s are constants (see Table 1).

The pressure developed by each OHC (P_{ohc}) is obtained from the spring properties of the OHC [6]. Let's define $\gamma_{\text{ohc}}(x)$ as the OHC effective index. It represents the effective distribution of the OHCs along the cochlear partition. Therefore, the OHC pressure is obtained by

$$P_{\text{ohc}}(x,t)=\gamma_{\text{ohc}}(x)\cdot K_{\text{ohc}}(x)\cdot\left[\xi_{\text{ohc}}(x,t)-\Delta l_{\text{ohc}}(x,t)\right], \tag{7}$$

where K_{ohc} is the OHC's stiffness (Table 1). A cochlea with no active OHC is obtained by $\gamma_{\text{ohc}}(x)=0$, whereas $0.5\le\gamma_{\text{ohc}}(x)\le 0.6$ yielded an optimal cochlea that best fits physiological data [13].

The ear model described by Eqs. (1)–(7) is solved by applying initial and boundary conditions. The boundary conditions are

$$\left.\begin{aligned}&\left.\frac{\partial P(x,t)}{\partial x}\right|_{x=0}=2\rho C_{\text{ow}}\frac{\partial^2\xi_{\text{ow}}(t)}{\partial t^2}\\ &P(L_{\text{co}},t)=0\end{aligned}\right\}, \tag{8}$$

where L_{co}=3.5 cm is the cochlear length, ξ_{ow} is the oval window displacement, and C_{ow} is the coupling factor of the oval window to the perilymph. In order to obtain ξ_{ow}, the middle ear model was applied [29] as expressed by the following differential equation:

$$\frac{d^2\xi_{\text{ow}}(t)}{d^2t}+\gamma_{\text{OW}}\cdot\frac{d\xi_{\text{ow}}(t)}{dt}+\omega_{\text{OW}}^2\xi_{\text{OW}}(t)=\frac{1}{\sigma_{\text{OW}}}\left[P(o,t)+\Gamma_{\text{me}}P_{\text{in}}(t)\right], \tag{9}$$

where σ_{ow} is the oval window areal density, γ_{ow} is the oval window resistance, and ω_{ow} is the oval window resonance frequency. The mechanical gain of the ossicles is denoted by Γ_{me} (see Table 1). $P_{\text{in}}(t)$ is the input acoustic stimulus.

The initial conditions are

$$\left.\begin{aligned}&\xi_{\text{bm}}(x,0)=\left.\frac{\partial\xi_{\text{bm}}(x,t)}{\partial t}\right|_{t=0}=0;\quad \xi_{\text{tm}}(x,0)=\left.\frac{\partial\xi_{\text{tm}}(x,t)}{\partial t}\right|_{t=0}=0;\quad \xi_{\text{ow}}(0)=\left.\frac{\mathrm{d}\xi_{\text{ow}}(t)}{\mathrm{d}t}\right|_{t=0}=0\\ &\psi_{\text{ohc}}(x,0)=\psi_0\end{aligned}\right\}. \tag{10}$$

http://dx.doi.org/10.5772/61189

Parameter	Value	Description
A	0.5	Cross-sectional area of the cochlea scalae $[\text{cm}^2]$
ρ	1	Perilymph density $[\text{g/cm}^3]$
β	0.003	Width of the basilar membrane [cm]
L_{co}	3.5	Cochlear length [cm]
K_{bm}	$1.282 \cdot 10^4 e^{-3x}$	Basilar membrane stiffness per unit area $[\text{g/cm}^2/\text{s}^2]$
R_{bm}	$0.25 \cdot e^{-0.6x}$	Basilar membrane damping per unit area $[\text{g/cm}^2/\text{s}]$
M_{bm}	$1.286 \cdot 10^{-6}$	Basilar membrane mass per unit area $[\text{g/cm}^2]$
K_{tm}	$3.97 \cdot 10^5 e^{-3x}$	Tectorial membrane stiffness per unit area $[\text{g/cm}^2/\text{s}^2]$
R_{tm}	$0.25 \cdot e^{-0.6x}$	Tectorial membrane damping per unit area $[\text{g/cm}^2/\text{s}]$
M_{tm}	0	Tectorial membrane mass per unit area $[\text{g/cm}^2]$
K_{ohc}	$400 \cdot e^{-3x}$	Outer hair cell membrane's stiffness $[\text{g/s}^2]$
α_s	10^{-6}	Peak to peak electromotility displacement [cm]
$1/\alpha_l$	$2 \cdot 10^{-6}$	Reference electromotility voltage [V]
ω_{ohc}	$2 \cdot \pi \cdot 1000$	Outer hair cell cutoff frequency [rad/s]
ψ_0	$-70 \cdot 10^{-3}$	Perilymph resting potential [V]
η	$3.14 \cdot 10^9$	[V/cm/s]
ω_{ow}	$2 \cdot \pi \cdot 1500$	Oval window cutoff frequency [Hz]
σ_{ow}	0.5	Oval window aerial density $[\text{g/cm}^2]$
γ_{ow}	$2 \cdot 10^4$	Oval window resistance $[1/s]$
C_{ow}	$6 \cdot 10^{-3}$	Coupling of oval window to perilymph [none]
Γ_{me}	21.4	Mechanical gain of ossicles [none]
η_{AC}	1	IHC AC coupling [V/s/cm]
η_{DC}	100	IHC DC coupling [V/cm]
Δ	$2 \cdot 10^{-3}$	IHC integration time [s]
A_{ihc}	1	AN coupling [spikes/s/V]
$\lambda_{\text{spont}}^{\text{H}}$	60	High spontaneous rate [spikes/s]
$\lambda_{\text{spont}}^{\text{M}}$	3	Medium spontaneous rate [spikes/s]
$\lambda_{\text{spont}}^{\text{L}}$	0.1	Low spontaneous rate [spikes/s]
λ_{sat}	500	Saturation rate [spikes/s]
A_{H}	70	Effective level threshold for high spontaneous rate [dB]
A_{M}	50	Effective level threshold for medium spontaneous rate [dB]
A_{L}	30	Effective level threshold for low spontaneous rate [dB]

Table 1. List of model parameters

2.1. Simulation results: The effect of outer hair cells loss

The above cochlear model was solved in the time domain by implementing a parallel algorithm on a commodity graphics processor unit (GPU) [14].The output of the model is the BM velocity ($\xi_{bm}(x, t)$) as a response to an acoustic stimulus $P_{in}(t)$.

Figure 3 represents the basilar membrane velocity relative to the input level at two points along the cochlear partition. The response was obtained by applying the model for a set of simple tones $P_0 \sin(2\pi f t)$ with a frequency of 100 Hz$< f <$8 kHz at different levels $0<P_0 \leq 120$ dB SPL. The gain plotted in Figure 3 was derived by $|\xi_{bm}(x)|/P_0$, where x=0.67 cm from the stapes (Figure 3A) and x=1.8 cm from the stapes (Figure 3B). Each solid line was obtained from a different level for a normal cochlea ($\gamma_{ohc}(x)$=0.5). The broken line represents an abnormal cochlea with 100% OHC loss, which was derived by the model by substituting $\gamma_{ohc}(x)$=0. For the normal cochlea, the maximum sensitivity at x=0.67 cm from the stapes (Figure 3A) was obtained when the stimulus was at 4 kHz and 0 dB SPL. The sensitivity is reduced with the increase in the input level, and the maximum sensitivity was shifted to a lower frequency (about 1 kHz). These results are in agreement with experimental results [30]. Figure 3B represents a characteristic frequency of 1 kHz that yielded wider responses as a function of frequency for all input levels. However, the gain of the damaged cochlea (broken line in Figure 3) was independent of the input level at both locations. When substituting $\gamma_{ohc}(x)$=0 in the cochlear model's equations, the nonlinear terms are zeroed and the model becomes linear.

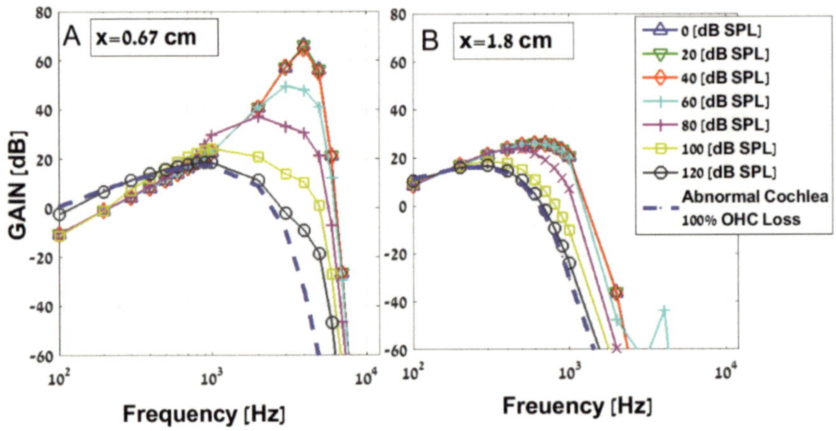

Figure 3. Derivation of the basilar membrane gain ($|\xi_{bm}(x_0)|/P_0$) as a function of input frequency at two locations along the cochlear partition: x = 0.67 cm from the stapes (A) and x = 1.8 cm from the stapes (B). Each solid line represents a different input level and a normal cochlea (γ_{ohc}=0.5). The broken line represents a damaged cochlea (γ_{ohc}=0). A similar gain was obtained for all input levels.

Figure 5 represents the relative BM velocity obtained by the model when the Hebrew word "SHEN" was introduced. The input word is presented in Figure 4 as a function of time (upper panel) and by its spectrogram (lower panel).

The absolute BM velocity in dB is presented in a color-coded two-dimensional image, whose x-axis represents the poststimulus time in milliseconds with its y-axis representing the distance from the stapes in cm. There are four images in Figure 5. The images in the left column represent a relative low input level (20 dB SPL), while the images in the right column represent an input level of 70 dB SPL. The upper panels represent a damaged cochlea with a 98% OHC loss (γ_{ohc}=0.01), while the lower panels represent a normal cochlea (γ_{ohc}=0.5). The difference between the normal and the damaged cochleae is clearly demonstrated in Figure 5 in both levels. In the damaged cochlea, the low-level stimulus yielded a BM vibration, which most likely will not be sufficient to evoke the neural response. Note that the maximum difference in the BM velocity between the normal and the damaged cochlea in response to the low-level stimuli is almost 40 dB. However, the maximum response between the two cochleae for the 70 dB input level is only 6 dB. This difference was induced by the nonlinear properties of the OHCs in the normal cochlea.

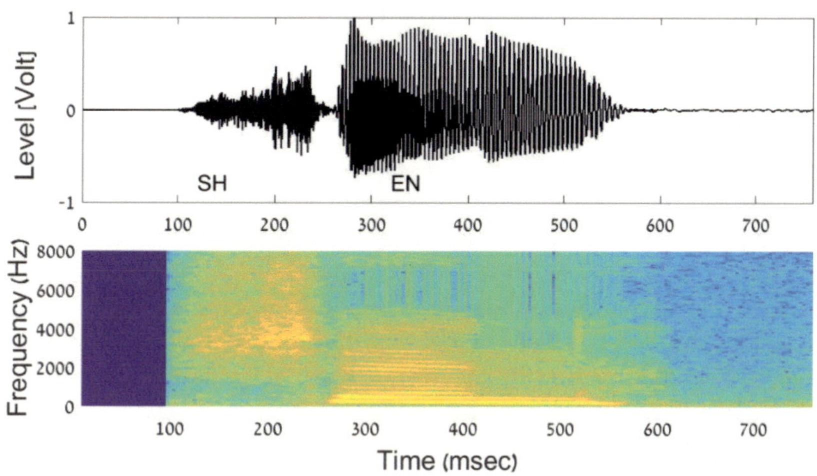

Figure 4. The Hebrew word "SHEN" pronounced by a female speaker. The sound pressure as a function of time (upper panel) and the correspondent spectrogram (lower panel).

The BM velocity in response to the consonant "sh" is very different in the four images in Figure 5. The maximum response was shifted toward the stapes when the amplitude was increased in the normal cochlea. In response to the high level stimuli, the maximum BM velocity obtained was closer to the stapes in the damaged cochlea than in the normal one.

3. Model of the Inner hair cell—auditory nerve synapse

The basilar membrane motion is transformed into neural spikes of the auditory nerve by the inner hair cells. The deflection of the hair-cell stereocilia opens mechanically gated ion channels that allow any small, positively charged ions (primarily potassium and calcium) to enter the cell [31]. Unlike many other electrically active cells, the hair cell itself does not fire an action

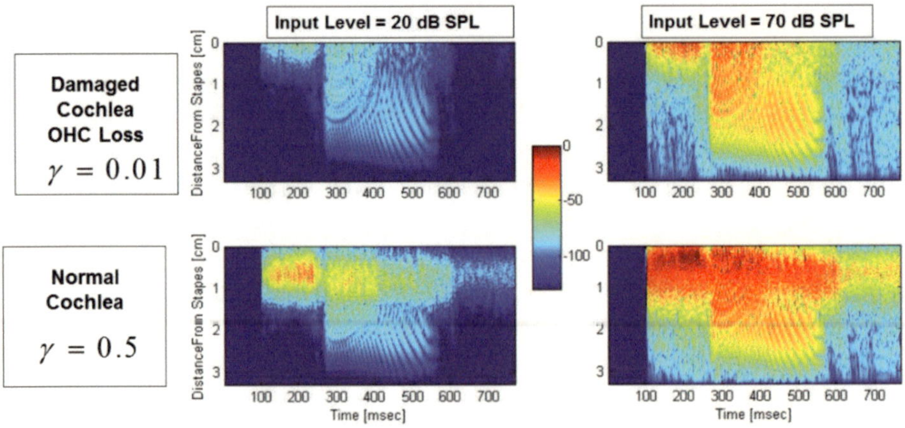

Figure 5. Relative BM velocity as a function of time along the cochlear partition as a response to the word "SHEN." The upper panels represent a damaged cochlea with outer hair cells loss and the lower panels represent a normal cochlea.

potential. Instead, the influx of positive ions from the endolymph in the scala media depolarizes the cell, resulting in a receptor potential. This receptor potential opens voltage-gated calcium channels; calcium ions then enter the cell and trigger the release of neurotransmitters at the basal end of the cell. The neurotransmitters diffuse across the narrow space between the hair cell and a nerve terminal, where they then bind to receptors and thus trigger action potentials in the nerve. In this way, the mechanical sound signal is converted into an electrical nerve signal. The IHCs chronically leak Ca^{+2}. This leakage causes a tonic release of neurotransmitter to the synapses. It is thought that this tonic release is what allows the hair cells to respond so quickly to mechanical stimuli. The quickness of the hair cell response may also be due to that fact that it can increase the amount of neurotransmitter release in response to a change as little as 100 μV in membrane potential.

Many models were developed for explaining the IHC's transduction abilities [16, 32, 33]. Some models focused on possible mechanisms for adaptation [17, 34–36]. Others were concerned with the biophysics of hair cells [37, 38] or the mechanoelectric transduction process [39].

One commonly simplified modeling approach to explain the IHC's role in the auditory system posits a nonlinear system that combines AC and DC responses followed by a random generator that creates spike trains [7, 16, 17, 40]. The model presented in this chapter is consistent with these principles.

The BM displacement stimulates the IHC cilia to move, its velocity ξ_{ihc} corresponding to the BM velocity (ξ_{bm}) by a nonlinear function, e.g.,

$$\dot{\xi}_{\text{ihc}} = \alpha_1 \tanh\left(\alpha_2 \cdot \dot{\xi}_{\text{bm}}\right) \approx \alpha_1 \cdot \left[\alpha_2 \cdot \dot{\xi}_{\text{bm}} - \frac{\left(\alpha_2 \cdot \dot{\xi}_{\text{bm}}\right)^3}{3} + \frac{2\left(\alpha_2 \cdot \dot{\xi}_{\text{bm}}\right)^5}{15} - \dots\right]. \tag{11}$$

Since the BM displacement in this model is nonlinear as described by the mechanical model above, we ignore the nonlinear terms in Eq. (11) and assume that $\alpha_1 \cdot \alpha_2 = 1$; therefore, $\xi_{\text{ihc}} \approx \xi_{\text{bm}}$.

The mechanoelectrical receptors that are located in the IHC membrane yield an increase in the electrical potential (ψ_{ihc}) of the IHC membrane. A common modeling approach for the IHC's role in the auditory system is based on a nonlinear system that combines AC and DC responses [7, 40]. The DC level represents the firing responses without any synchrony to the input stimuli and the AC level represents the synchronized firing response (typical at low frequencies). The DC component includes a high-pass filter followed by a moving average filter of 2 ms long; the AC component consists of a low-pass filter. In order to account for physiological observations that demonstrated a reduction in synchronization as the frequency of the stimulus increases[41], we chose a low-pass filter with a cutoff frequency of 1000 Hz, with a slope of 30 dB/decade. In practice, ψ_{ihc} is obtained by

$$\psi_{\text{ihc}}(x,t) = e^{\gamma_{\text{ihc}}(x)} \cdot \left\{ \eta_{\text{AC}} \cdot \dot{\xi}_{\text{ihc}}(x,t) * h_{\text{ihc}}(t) + \eta_{\text{DC}} \cdot \int_{t-\Delta}^{t} \left\{ \dot{\xi}_{\text{ihc}}(x,t) * \left[1 - h_{\text{ihc}}(t)\right] \right\}^2 dt \right\}, \tag{12}$$

where x represents the location of the IHC along the cochlear partition, $h_{\text{ihc}}(t)$ is the impulse response of the low-pass filter that represents the IHC response, and η_{AC}, η_{DC}, and Δ are constants (see Table 1). The parameter $\gamma_{\text{ihc}}(x)$ represents the IHC efficiency index. It was defined as a function of x, to allow variability in IHC efficiency along the cochlear partition. For normal cochlea, we chose $\gamma_{\text{ihc}}(x)=8$, which was found to match experimental data. The efficiency of the IHC is reduced with a decrease of $\gamma_{\text{ihc}}(x)$.

This IHC receptor potential opens voltage-gated calcium channels; calcium ions then enter the cell and trigger the release of neurotransmitters at the basal end of the cell. The neurotransmitters diffuse across the narrow space between the hair cell and a nerve terminal where they then bind to receptors and thus trigger action potentials in the nerve.

The neural activity in the auditory system is irregular since a specific neuron might respond with a single spike or several spikes to a given stimuli [42]. The origin of the stochastic activity of neurons is poorly understood. This activity results in both intrinsic noise sources that generate stochastic behavior on the level of the neuronal dynamics and extrinsic sources that arise from network effects and synaptic transmission [43]. Another source of noise that is specific to neurons arises from the finite number of ion channels in a neuronal membrane patch [31, 44].

There are a number of different ways that have emerged to describe the stochastic properties of neural activity. One possible approach relates to the train of spikes as a stochastic point process. For example, in their earlier studies, Alaoglu and Smith [45] and Rodieck et al. [46] suggested that the spontaneous activity of the cochlear nucleus can be described as a homogeneous Poisson process. Further investigations of the auditory system described the neural response as a nonhomogeneous Poisson point process (NHPP) whose instantaneous rate depends on the input stimuli [47, 48].

In the present chapter, we relate to the neural activity as NHHP, and thus only the instantaneous rate (IR) should be extracted. In order to derive IR, we use the Weber–Fechner law, which describes the relationship between the magnitude of a physical stimulus and the intensity or strength that people feel. This kind of relationship can be described by a differential equation:

$$dP = K\frac{dS}{S}$$

where dP is the differential change in perception, dS is the differential increase in the stimulus, and S is the stimulus at the instant. Integrating the above equation reveals $P = k \cdot \ln S + C$. Let us define $\lambda_{AN}(x, t)$ as the IR obtained by the auditory fiber attached to location x along the cochlear partition, and let us assume that it relates to the perception of the physical parameter. On the other hand, $\psi_{ihc}(x, t)$, the IHC electrical potential corresponds to the stimulus. Therefore, by applying the Weber–Fechner law, we obtained the relationship $\lambda_{AN}(x, t) = \ln(\psi_{ihc}(x, t)) + C$. However, the AN's IR should satisfy the following conditions: $0 < \lambda_{spont} \leq \lambda_{AN}(x, t) \leq \lambda_{sat}$, where λ_{spont} and λ_{sat} are the spontaneous and saturation rates of the AN, respectively. Therefore, $\lambda_{AN}(x, t)$ is obtained by

$$\lambda_{AN}(x,t) = \min\left\{\lambda_{sat}, \max\left\{\lambda_{spont}, A_{ihc} \cdot \ln\left(1 + u(\psi_{ihc}(x,t))\right)\right\}\right\}, \tag{13}$$

where u is the step function and A_{ihc} is a constant (see Table 1).

In general, the auditory nerve response is divided into three types of fibers according to their spontaneous rates: a high spontaneous rate (HSR) that usually codes low-level stimuli, a medium spontaneous rate (MSR), and a high spontaneous rate (LSR) that generally codes high level stimuli. In order to include all types of auditory nerves, we substitute in Eq. (13) the relevant constants $\left[\lambda_{spont}^{(H)}, A_H; \lambda_{spont}^{(M)}, A_M; \lambda_{spont}^{(L)}, A_L\right]$ for the HSR, MSR, and LSR that yield the instantaneous rates $\left[\lambda_{AN}^{(H)}(x, t), \lambda_{AN}^{(M)}(x, t), \lambda_{AN}^{(L)}(x, t)\right]$, respectively. The different types of ANs are distributed uniformly along the cochlear partition, where the most frequent fibers are those with a low spontaneous rate (about 60%).

The IRs (spikes per second) for the LSR fibers, $\lambda_{AN}^{(L)}(x, t)$, as a response to the Hebrew word "SHEN" are exhibited in Figure 6 by color-coded images as a function of time (x-axis) and along the cochlear partition (y-axis). The basilar membrane velocity as a response to this word was shown in Figure 5 for two different levels. In Figure 6, the response to the high level stimulus (70 dB SPL) is displayed. Four images are presented in Figure 6, each representing a different type of cochlea. Each cochlea is defined by the two indices, γ_{ohc} and γ_{ihc}, which represent the efficiency of the OHC and IHC, respectively. In this example, both indices were constant along the cochlear partition. For normal cochlea, we chose γ_{ohc}=0.5 and γ_{ihc}=8 ; these values exhibit the best fit to experimental data [13].

The upper-left image in Figure 6 represents a normal cochlea (γ_{ohc}=0.5; γ_{ihc}=8). The upper-right image corresponds to a cochlea with intact OHC but with 25% IHC loss (γ_{ihc}=6). A clear reduction in the instantaneous rate is shown. The maximum instantaneous rate was reduced from 160 spikes/s in the normal cochlea to 100 in the damaged one. Moreover, in the damaged cochlea, about 25% more instances (time and location along the cochlear partition) reached the spontaneous rate 0.1 spikes/s relative to the normal cochlea.

The two lower images in Figure 6 represent cochleae with 98% OHC loss (γ_{ohc}=0.01). The BM response was changed as Figure 5 shows. Thus, the reduction in the instantaneous rate corresponds entirely to the decrease in BM velocity when the cochlea has intact IHCs (lower-left image). For a cochlea with both OHC and IHC loss (lower-right image), the instantaneous rate was reduced because of both losses. The response to the high frequencies that correspond to the syllable "SH" almost vanished.

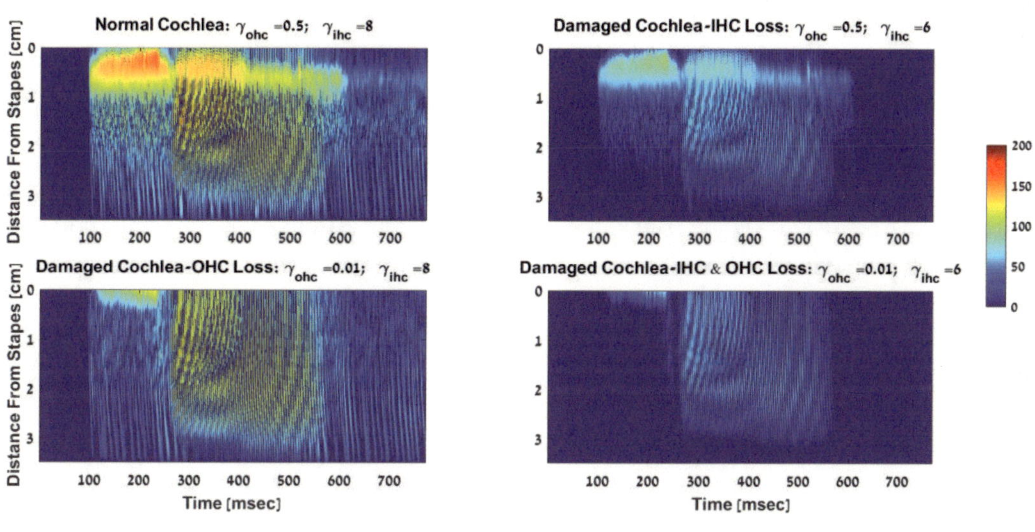

Figure 6. Derived instantaneous rates as a response to the Hebrew word "SHEN" at 70 dB SPL. Each panel represents a different type of ear. The upper-left panel represents a normal cochlea. The upper-right panel represents a cochlea with IHC loss. The lower-left panel represents a cochlea with OHC loss and the lower-right panel represents both IHC and OHC loss.

4. Threshold estimation based on the auditory nerve

The hearing threshold, defined as the lowest threshold of acoustic pressure sensation, is usually determined by quantitative psychoacoustical experiments in which the human ability to detect the smallest difference in the stimulus' physical property is obtained. This difference is referred to as a just-noticeable difference (JND). In such experiments, a subject must distinguish between two close time (t) dependent stimuli: $s(t, \alpha)$ and $s(t, \alpha + \Delta\alpha)$, where α is a given physical property. The JND(α) will be the minimum $\Delta\alpha$ a person can perceive. The parameter α represents any physical property of the stimulus that can be measured such as frequency or level in monaural stimulus.

Comparing the behavioral JND and the neural activity is possible if one assumes that the neural system estimates the measured parameters. Siebert [18] obtained such a comparison when the JND of a single tone's frequency and level was compared to the neural activity of the auditory nerve. Siebert's findings were based on the assumption that the auditory nerve (AN) response behaves as an NHPP, and the brain acts as an unbiased optimal estimator of the physical parameters. Thus, the JND is equal to the standard deviation of the estimated parameter and can be derived by lower bounds such as the Cramer–Rao lower bound. Heinz et al. [49]) generalized Sibert's results to a larger range of frequencies and levels.

In a psychoacoustical JND experiment, the yielded JND value is obtained when $d'=1$, which is expressed by:

$$d' = \frac{E\left[\hat{\alpha} \mid \alpha^*\right] - E\left[\hat{\alpha} \mid \left(\alpha^* + \Delta\alpha\right)\right]}{std\left(\hat{\alpha} \mid \alpha^*\right)} = \frac{\Delta\alpha}{std\left(\hat{\alpha} \mid \alpha^*\right)}, \tag{14}$$

where $E[\hat{\alpha} \mid \alpha^*] = \alpha^*$, α^* is the true value of α, and $\hat{\alpha}$ is the estimated value of α. Therefore, $d'=1$, yields the relations $\Delta\alpha = std(\hat{\alpha} \mid \alpha^*)$, which implies

$$\text{JND}\left(\alpha^*\right) = std\left(\hat{\alpha} \middle| \alpha^*\right). \tag{15}$$

When the estimation is based on neural activity that behaves as NHPP, there are two possible ways to analyze the performance. The first way is referred to as "rate coding" (RA), which means that the performance is analyzed on the basis of the number of spikes. The second way is referred as "all information coding" (AI), indicating that in addition to the number of spikes in the interval, the timing of the discharge spikes is considered as well.

Let us define $N(0, T)$ as the random variable that represents the number of spikes in the time interval $[0, T]$. For the RA coding, the probability density function (pdf) of getting n spikes in the time interval of length T is obtained by

$$P_{\text{RA}}\left(N\left(0,T\right) = n\right) = \frac{1}{n!}\left[\int_0^T \lambda\left(t,\alpha\right)dt\right]^n \exp\left\{-\int_0^T \lambda\left(t,\alpha\right)dt\right\}, \tag{16}$$

where $\lambda(t, \alpha)$ is the instantaneous rate of the nerve fiber that depends on both the time t and the physical parameter α. Given the RA pdf (Eq. (16)), the resulting Cramer–Rao lower bound (CRLB) is obtained by [50]

$$\mathrm{CRLB}_{\mathrm{RA}}\left(\alpha^*\right)=\left\{\frac{T}{\bar{\lambda}\left(\alpha^*\right)}\left[\left.\frac{\partial\bar{\lambda}(\alpha)}{\partial\alpha}\right|_{\alpha=\alpha^*}\right]^2\right\}^{-\frac{1}{2}} \tag{17}$$

where $\bar{\lambda}(\alpha)=\frac{1}{T}\int_0^T\lambda(t, \alpha)dt$ is the average rate.

For the AI coding, the probability density function of getting n successive neural spikes at a set of time instances is $[t_1, t_2, \ldots, t_n]$, where $0\le t_1<t_2<\ldots<t_n\le T$ is obtained by

$$P_{\mathrm{AI}}\left(N(0,T=n);t_1,\ldots,t_n\right)=\frac{1}{n!}\prod_{k=1}^{n}\lambda\left(t_k,\alpha\right)\exp\left\{-\int_0^T\lambda\left(t,\alpha\right)dt\right\}. \tag{18}$$

The resulting CRLB was derived by Bar David [51], which yields

$$\mathrm{CRLB}_{\mathrm{AI}}\left(\alpha^*\right)=\left\{\int_0^T\frac{1}{\lambda\left(t,\alpha^*\right)}\left[\left.\frac{\partial\lambda\left(t,\alpha\right)}{\partial\alpha}\right|_{\alpha=\alpha^*}\right]^2dt\right\}^{-\frac{1}{2}}. \tag{19}$$

In every unbiased system, the following relations hold:

$$std\left(\left[\hat{\alpha}\middle|\alpha^*\right]\right)\ge\mathrm{CRLB}_{\mathrm{RATE}}\left(\alpha^*\right)\ge\mathrm{CRLB}_{\mathrm{AI}}\left(\alpha^*\right). \tag{20}$$

In an optimal unbiased system, the standard deviation of the estimator can achieve the lower bounds. Since $\mathrm{JND}(\alpha^*)=std(\hat{\alpha}\mid\alpha^*)$ (Eq. 15), $\mathrm{JND}(\alpha^*)$ can be estimated by calculating $\mathrm{CRLB}_{\mathrm{RA}}(\alpha^*)$ or $\mathrm{CRLB}_{\mathrm{AI}}(\alpha^*)$. Comparing the estimated thresholds to experimental results can resolve the question whether the brain estimates the auditory thresholds according to RA or AI coding.

In order to apply the above-mentioned method for determining the auditory threshold, we should consider the responses of all 30,000 AN fibers that innervate each ear. Since the AN fibers are statistically independent [2], the d' theorem can be applied, which yields

$$(d')^2 = \sum_{m=1}^{M} (d_m')^2, \tag{21}$$

where M is the number of nerve fibers and d_m' is the d' (Eq. 14) that was derived for the mth fiber. Moreover,

$$std(\hat{\alpha} \mid \alpha^*) = 1 \Big/ \sqrt{\sum_{m=1}^{M} \{std_m(\hat{\alpha} \mid \alpha^*)\}^{-2}}, \tag{22}$$

where $std_m(\hat{\alpha} \mid \alpha^*)$ is the standard deviation of the estimator obtained by the mth fiber. Since the threshold is obtained when $d'=1$, it implies that in an optimal system,

$$JND(\alpha^*) = 1 \Big/ \sqrt{\sum_{m=1}^{M} \{CRLB_m(\alpha^*)\}^{-2}}, \tag{23}$$

where $\mathrm{CRLB}_m(\alpha^*)$ is the CRLB of the mth fiber.

Let us define the number of fibers attached to each location along the cochlear partition as $M(x)$. Thus, $\sum_{x \notin [0, L_{co}]} M(x) = 30,000$, where L_{CO} is the cochlear length. For every location, three IRs were derived $\lambda_{AN}^{(H)}(x,t)$, $\lambda_{AN}^{(M)}(x,t)$, $\lambda_{AN}^{(L)}(x,t)$ (Eq. 13), which correspond to the HSR, MSR, and LSR fibers, respectively. They are distributed uniformly along the cochlear partition with corresponding weights $[w_L, w_M, w_H]$ (see Table 1). Therefore,

$$\mathrm{JND}(\alpha^*) = \frac{1}{\sqrt{F_L + F_M + F_H}}, \tag{24}$$

where

$$\left.\begin{aligned} F_L &= \sum_{x \in [0, L_{CO}]} \sum_{m=1}^{w_L \cdot M(x)} \{\mathrm{CRLB}_m^{(L)}(\alpha^*)\}^{-2} \\ F_M &= \sum_{x \in [0, L_{CO}]} \sum_{m=1}^{w_M \cdot M(x)} \{\mathrm{CRLB}_m^{(M)}(\alpha^*)\}^{-2} \\ F_H &= \sum_{x \in [0, L_{CO}]} \sum_{m=1}^{w_H \cdot M(x)} \{\mathrm{CRLB}_m^{(H)}(\alpha^*)\}^{-2} \end{aligned}\right\}. \tag{25}$$

Replacing *CRLB* in Eq. (24) with the corresponding $CRLB_{RA}(\alpha^*)$ or $CRLB_{AI}(\alpha^*)$, $JND(\alpha^*)$is estimated by either RATE or AI coding.

4.1. Simulation results: rate or all information?

In order to calculate both $CRLB_{RATE}(\alpha^*)$ and $CRLB_{AI}(\alpha^*)$, the derivative of the instantaneous rate should be derived. We have used the following approximation:

$$\partial\lambda(t,\alpha)/\partial\alpha\big|_{\alpha=\alpha^*} \approx \frac{\lambda(t,\alpha^* + \Delta\alpha) - \lambda(t,\alpha^*)}{\Delta\alpha}. \tag{26}$$

Therefore, in deriving $JND(\alpha^*)$ for any stimulus $s(t, \alpha^*)$, the IRs for both stimuli $s(t, \alpha^*)$ and $s(t, \alpha^* + \Delta\alpha)$ should be calculated. Two types of thresholds will be presented for tones in quiet and in the presence of noise. The quiet threshold was derived by substituting $\alpha^*=0$ that yielded $\lambda(t, \alpha^*)=\lambda_{spont}$. For the thresholds in the presence of noise, $s(t, \alpha^*)$ is equal to the noise, and $s(t, \alpha^* + \Delta\alpha)$ is equal to the noise +tone with a level of $\Delta\alpha$.

We have calculated the amplitude thresholds as a function of frequency while using both types of coding, RA and AI. The derived thresholds are shown in Figure 7 along with normal equal-loudness-level contour at threshold (ISO 226:2003) [52]. The rate coding successfully predicts the ISO 226 standard while the AI coding yielded performances that are better by a few decibels. This difference was not sufficient for deciding what type of coding is used by the brain in order to determine the absolute thresholds. Deriving the thresholds in the presence of noise revealed a more significant difference between the two types of coding.

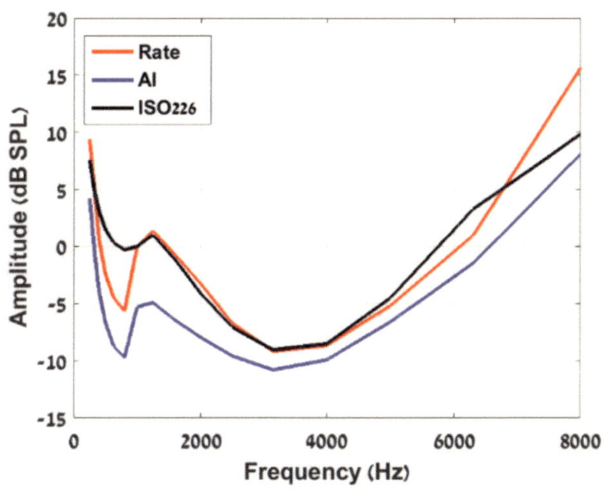

Figure 7. Estimated thresholds as a function of frequency obtained by a normal cochlea according to both rate and AI coding along with normal equal-loudness-level contour at threshold (ISO 226:2003).

In order to present the threshold of tones in the presence of noise, the smallest perceivable difference is presented in terms of difference limen (DL), which are defined as

$$DL = 10 \cdot \log_{10}\left(1 + \frac{\Delta\alpha}{\alpha^*}\right), \tag{27}$$

where α^* corresponds to the noise level in Volts and $\Delta\alpha$ is the derived *JND* of the tone level in Volts. Figure 8 represents the DL of tones as a function of noise level for different frequencies. The noise was Gaussian white noise. The tone thresholds were derived by both types of coding (RA and AI), and they are presented in Figure 8 along with experimental data from Miller [54, 55]. Both types of coding succeeded in predicting the experimental result that the dependence of DL on noise level is independent of the tone's frequency. However, only RA coding yielded similar values of DL as a function of noise level. The AI coding revealed DL values that were lower by order of magnitude than the experimental result. This result convinced us that the brain is using rate coding in order to estimate tone amplitude.

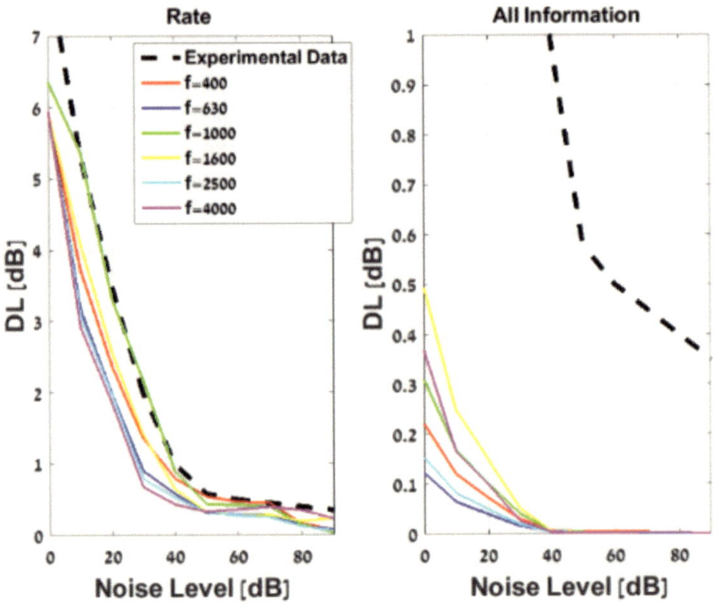

Figure 8. DL as a function of noise level as obtained by a normal cochlea according to both rate (left panel) and AI (right panel) coding. Each color represents a different frequency. The black broken line was replotted from [55].

4.2. Simulation results: Abnormal ears

Audiograms of the hearing impaired were estimated by subtracting the threshold of the damaged ear from the threshold defined by the equal loudness at threshold [52]. The estimated audiograms of different types of pathologies are shown in Figure 9. In all the estimated audiograms, we assumed that both IHC and OHC loss were uniform along the cochlear partition, which implies that $\gamma_{ihc}(x)$=const. and $\gamma_{ohc}(x)$=const.

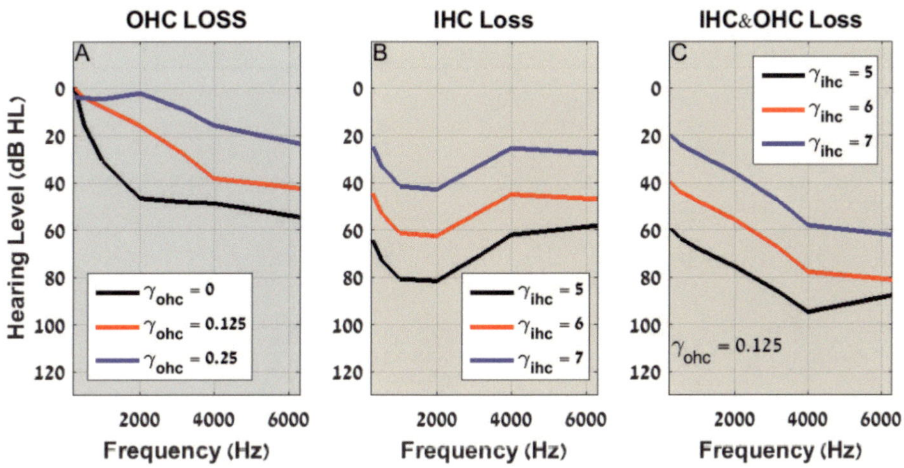

Figure 9. Estimated audiograms for different type of pathologies. Panel A represents cochleae with different degrees of OHC loss and intact IHC. Panel B represents cochleae with different degrees of IHC loss and intact OHC. Panel C represents cochlea with both IHC and OHC loss.

Three audiograms are exhibited in panel A of Figure 9. They were obtained with γ_{ihc}=8 (the normal value) and three values of γ_{ohc}=0, 0.125, 0.25 that represent 100%, 75%, and 50% of OHC loss, respectively. Due to OHC loss of 50%, no hearing loss was obtained up to 2 kHz. With 100% OHC loss, the estimated audiogram revealed a maximum hearing loss of about 60 dB at 6 kHz. Panel B of Figure 9 represents cochleae with no OHC loss (γ_{ohc}=0.5) but with different degrees of IHC loss, γ_{ihc}=5, 6, 7, which represents 37.5%, 25%, and 12.5% of IHC efficiency. Reduction in IHC efficiency caused a maximum hearing loss at 1000–2000 Hz. A combination of IHC and OHC loss is probably a more common pathology; an example of its effect is shown in Figure 9C. It represents cochleae with 75% OHC loss (γ_{ohc}=0.125) and different degrees of IHC loss. The maximum hearing loss was obtained at 4 kHz. The estimated audiogram with γ_{ihc}=7 resembles a typical mild audiogram while the one with γ_{ihc}=5 resembles a typical severe audiogram.

The effect of background noise on the threshold to tones is demonstrated in Figure 10, where DL is plotted as a function of noise level for different frequencies. As a result of OHC loss, γ_{ohc}=0, and a significant increase in DL was yielded especially at high frequencies relative to normal cochlea. The combination of IHC and OHC loss caused an increase in DL at all frequencies. It seems that the effect of IHC loss causes an increase in DL at low frequencies below 1000 Hz. This result might explain the difficulties of people with mild hearing loss to understand speech in a noisy background. The information of speech sounds is mainly included in the low frequency range.

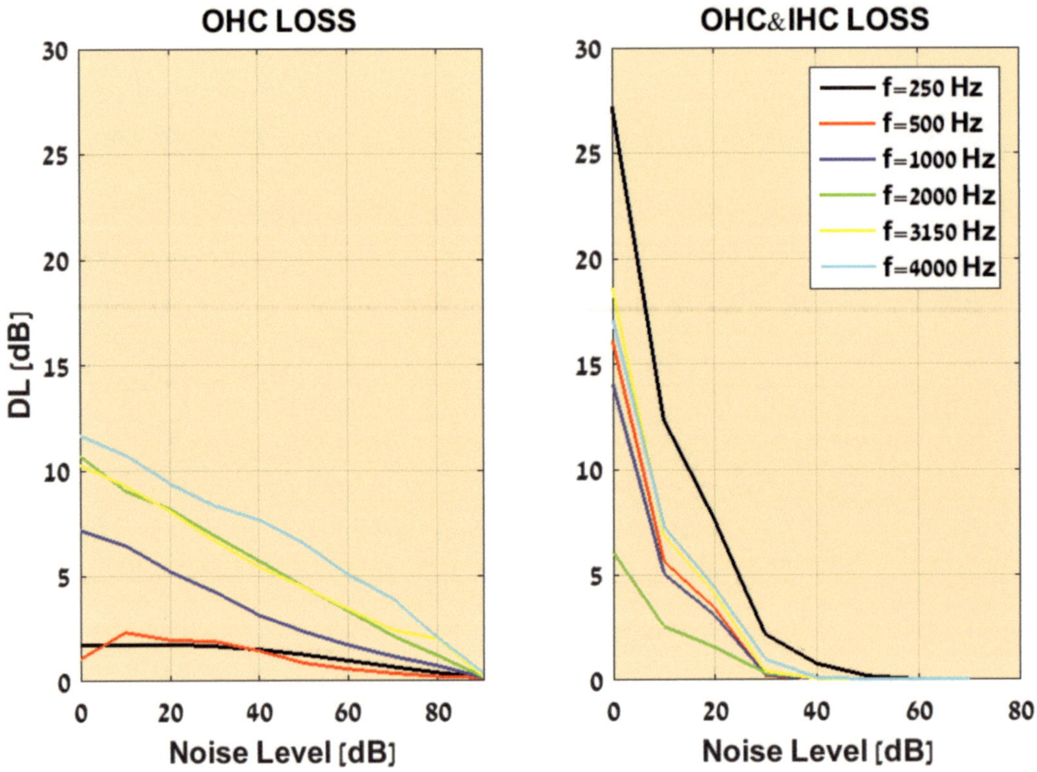

Figure 10. DL as a function of noise level as obtained by abnormal cochleae. Left panel represents a cochlea with 100% OHC loss (γ_{ohc}=0) and intact IHC. Right panel represents a cochlea with both IHC and OHC loss (γ_{ohc}=0.125; γ_{ihc}=6). Each color represents a different frequency.

5. Summary

In this study, a comprehensive model for the auditory system was introduced. It included a detailed, nonlinear time domain cochlear model with active outer hair cells that are driven by the tectorial membrane motion. Outer hair cell loss was indicated by an OHC efficiency index that could change along the cochlear partition. The second part of the model included a synaptic model that generates the auditory nerve's instantaneous rate as a response to basilar membrane motion and is affected by inner hair cell transduction efficiency. Since both inner and outer hair cell loss can be easily integrated in the model, the model is useful for demonstrating those pathologies.

In order to compare normal and abnormal human abilities to the model predictions, a comprehensive technique was introduced. It was based on the assumption that the brain behaves as an optimal processor and its task in JND experiments is to estimate physical parameters. The performance of the optimal processor can be derived by calculating its lower

http://dx.doi.org/10.5772/61189

bound. Since the neural activity was described as an NHPP, the Cramer–Rao lower bound was analytically derived for both rate and all information coding.

In this study, we have shown that the amplitude of tones in quiet and in the presence of background noise is most likely coded by the rate only. Pathological audiograms can be predicted by introducing reduced OHC and IHC efficiency indices. Moreover, the presence of noise causes a significant increase in DL. The effect of DL as a function of frequency depends on the type of hearing loss. In general, OHC loss mostly effects the high frequencies, while the effect of IHC loss is mostly expressed in the low frequencies.

The model presented in this paper can be used as a framework to explore different types of pathologies on the basis of audiograms obtained in quiet and in the presence of background noise.

Acknowledgements

This research was partially supported by the Israel Science Foundation grant no. 563/12. I want to express my great appreciation to my students who participated in this research over the years: Ram Krips, Azi Cohen, Vered Weiss, Noam Elbaum, Oren Cohen, Dan Mekrantz, Oded Barzely, Yaniv Halmut, and Tal Kalp.

Author details

Miriam Furst*

School of Electrical Engineering, Faculty of Engineering, Tel Aviv University, Tel Aviv, Israel

References

[1] Moore, B.C.J. (2007). Cochlear Hearing Loss. Wiley, West Sussex, United Kingdom.

[2] Heinz, M.G. (2010). Computational modeling of sensorineural hearing loss. In: Computational Models of the Auditory System, edited by R. Meddis, E.A. Lopez-Poveda, A.N. Popper, and R.R. Fay. Springer, New York, pp. 177–202.

[3] Jepsen, M.L., Ewert, S.D., and Dau, T. (2008). A computational model of human auditory signal processing and perception. J. Acoust. Soc. Am. 124, 422–438.

[4] Lopez-Poveda, E.A. and Meddis, R. (2001). A human nonlinear cochlear filterbank. J. Acoust. Soc. Am., 110, 3107–3118.

[5] Zilany, M.S.A., and Bruce, I.C. (2006). Modeling auditory-nerve responses for high sound pressure levels in the normal and impaired auditory periphery. J. Acoust. Soc. Am. 120: 1446–1466.

[6] Cohen A. and Furst M. (2004). Integration of outer hair cell activity in one-dimensional cochlear mode. J. Acoust. Soc. Am., 115:2185–2192.

[7] Carney L.H. (1993). A model for the responses of low-frequency auditory-nerve fibers in cat. J Acoust. Soc. Am. 93:401–417.

[8] Kates, J.M. (1991). A time-domain digital cochlear model. IEEE Trans. Signal Process. 39, 2573–2592.

[9] Goldstein, J.L. (1990). Modeling rapid waveform compression on the basilar membrane as multiple-bandpass-nonlinearity filtering. Hear. Res. 49, 39–60.

[10] Hopkins, K. and Moore, B.C.J (2011). The effects of age and cochlear hearing loss on temporal fine structure sensitivity, frequency selectivity, and speech reception in noise. J Acoust. Soc. Am. 130: 334–349.

[11] Jepsen, M.L. and Dau, T. (2011). Characterizing auditory processing and perception in individual listeners with sensorineural hearing loss. J. Acoust. Soc. Am., 129, 262–281.

[12] Furst, M. and Halmut, Y. (2006). Prediction for audiograms and otoacoustic emissions. In: Auditory Mechanisms: Processes and Models, edited by A.L. Nuttal, T. Ren, P. Gillespie, K. Grosh, and E. de Boer. World Scientific Publishing, pp. 384–385.

[13] Barzelay, O. and Furst, M. (2011). Time domain one-dimensional cochlear model with integrated tectorial membrane and outerhair cells. In: What Fire Is in Mine Ears Progress in Auditory Biomechanics, Vol 84, edited by C.A. Shera and E.S. Olson. American Institute of Physics, pp. 79–84.

[14] Sabo, D., Barzelay, O., Weiss, S., and Furst, M. (2014). Fast evaluation of a time-domain non-linear cochlear model on GPUs. J. Comput. Phys. 265: 97–113.

[15] Dau, T., Püschel, D., and Kohlrausch, A. (1996). A quantitative model of the effective signal processing in the auditory system. I. Model structure. J. Acoust. Soc. Am. 99, 3615–3622.

[16] Sumner, C., Lopez-Poveda, E., O'Mard, L., and Meddis, R.(2002). A revised model of the inner-hair cell and auditory-nerve complex. J. Acoust. Soc. Am. 111, 2178–2189.

[17] Zilany, M.S.A., Bruce, I.C., Nelson, P.C., and Carney, L.H. (2009). A phenomenological model of the synapse between the inner hair cell and auditory nerve: long-term adaptation with power-law. J. Acoust. Soc. Am. 126, 2390–2412.

[18] Siebert, W.M. (1970). Frequency discrimination in the auditory system: place or periodicity mechanism. Proc. IEEE 58, 723–730.

[19] Brownell, W.E., Bader, C.R., Bertrand D., and de Ribaupierre, I. (1985). Evoked mechanical responses of isolated cochlear outer hair cells. Science 227: 194–196.

[20] Zwislocki, J.J. (1950). Theory of the acoustical action of the cochlea. J. Acoust. Soc. Am. 22: 778–784.

[21] Zweig, G., Lipes, R., and Pierce, J.R. (1976). The cochlear compromise. J. Acoust. Soc. Am. 59: 975–982.

[22] Viergever, M.A. (1980). Mechanics of the inner ear a mathematical approach. Delft University of technology, Netherlands.

[23] Furst, M., Goldstein, J.L. (1982). A cochlear transmission line model compatible with psychophysics. J. Acoust. Soc. Am. 72: 717–726.

[24] Dallos, P.(2003). Organ of Corti Kinematics. J. Assoc. Res. Otolaryngol. 4: 416–421.

[25] Mountain, D.C. and Hubbard, A.E. (1995). Computational analysis of hair cell and auditory nerve processes. In: Auditory Computation, edited by H.L. Hawkins, T.A. McMullen, A.N. Popper, and R.R. Fay. Springer, pp. 121–156.

[26] Zheng, J., Madison, L.D., Oliver, D., Fakler, B., and Dallos, P. (2002). Prestin, the motor protein of outer hair cells. Audiol. Neurootol. 2002, 7: 9–12.

[27] He, D.Z.Z. and Dallos, P. (2000). Properties of voltage-dependent somatic stiffness of cochlear outer haircells. J. Assoc. Res. Otolaryngol. 1:64–81.

[28] Liu, Y.W. and Neely, S.T. (2009). Outer hair cell electromechanical properties in a nonlinear piezoelectric model. J. Acoust. Soc. Am. 126:751–761.

[29] Talmadge, C.L., Tubis, A., Long, G.L, and Piskorski, P. (1998). Modeling otoacoustic emission and hearing threshold fine structure. J. Acoust. Soc. Am. 104:1517–1543.

[30] Robles, L. and Ruggero, M.A. (2001). Mechanics of the mammalian cochlea. Physiol. Rev. 81:1305–1352.

[31] White, J.A., Rubinstein, J.T., and Kay, A.R. (2000). Channel noise in neurons. Trends Neurosci. 23: 131–137.

[32] Davis, H. (1965). A model for transducer action in the cochlea. Cold Spring Harb. Symp. Quant. Biol. 30, 181–189.

[33] Meddis, R., O'Mard, L.P., and Lopez-Poveda, E.A. (2001). A computational algorithm for computing nonlinear auditory frequency selectivity. J. Acoust. Soc. Am. 109: 2852–2861.

[34] Schroeder, M.R. and Hall, J.L. (1974). Model for mechanical to neural-transduction in the auditory receptor. J. Acoust. Soc. Am. 55: 1055–1060.

[35] Smith, R.L. and Brachman, M.L. (1982). Adaptation in auditory-nerve fibers: a revised model. Biol. Cybern. 44: 107–120.

[36] Meddis, R. (1986). Simulation of mechanical to neural transduction in the auditory receptor. J. Acoust. Soc. Am. 79: 702–711.

[37] Shamma, S.A., Chadwick, R.S., Wilbur, W.J., Morrish, K.A., and Rinzel,J.(1986). A biophysical model of the cochlear processing: intensity dependence of pure tone responses. J. Acoust. Soc. Am. 80: 133–145.

[38] Rattay, F., Gebeshuber, I.C., and Gitter, A.H. (1998). The mammalian auditory hair cell: a simple electric circuit model. J. Acoust. Soc. Am.103: 1558–1565.

[39] Corey, D.P., and Hudspeth, A.J. (1983). Kinetics of the receptor current in the bullfrog saccular hair-cells. J. Neurosci. 3: 962–976.

[40] Schoonhoven, R., Keijzer, J., Versnel, H., Prijs, V.F. (1993). A dual filter model describing single-fiber responses to clicks in the normal and noise-damaged cochlea. J. Acoust. Soc. Am. 95: 2104–2121.

[41] Palmer, A.M. and Russell, I.J. (1986). Phase-locking in the cochlear nerve of the guinea-pig and its relation to the receptor potential of inner hair-cells. Hear. Res. 24: 1–15.

[42] Kiang N.Y.S., Watanabe T., Thomas E.C., and Clark L.F. (1965). Discharge Patterns of Single Fibers in the Cat's Auditory Nerve. Cambridge MA, MIT press.

[43] Manwani, A. and Koch C. (1999). Detecting and estimating signals in noisy cable structures: I. neuronal noise sources. Neural Comput. 11: 1797–1829.

[44] Schneidman E., Freedman B., and Segev I. (1998). Channel stochasticity may be critical in determining the reliability and precision of spike timing. Neural Comput. 10: 1679–1703.

[45] Alaoglu, L. and Smith, N.M. Jr. (1938). Statistical theory of a scaling circuit. Phys. Rev. 53: 832 – 836.

[46] Rodieck, R.W., Kiang N.Y.-S., and Gerstein G.L. (1962). Some quantitative methods for the study of spontaneous activity of single neurons. Biophys. J. 2: 351–368.

[47] Gray, P.R. (1967). Conditional probability analyses of the spike activity of single neurons. Biophys. J. 10: 759–777.

[48] Rieke F., Warland D., van Steveninck R.D.R., and Bialek W. (1997). Spikes Exploring the Neural Code. MIT Press, Cambridge, Mass, USA.

[49] Heinz, M.G., Colburn, H.S., and Carney, L.H. (2001). Evaluating auditory performance limits: I. One-parameter discrimination using a computational model for the auditory nerve. Neural Comput. 13: 2273–2316.

[50] Snyder D.L. and Miller M.I. (1991). Random Point Processes in Time and Space. Springer-Verlag Berlin and Heidelberg GmbH & Co. K.

[51] Bar David, I. (1969). Communication under Poisson regime. IEEE Trans. Inf. Theory 15: 31–37.

[52] ISO226:2003:http://www.iso.org/iso/iso_catalogue/catalogue_tc/catalogue_detail.htm?csnumber=34222.

http://dx.doi.org/10.5772/61189

[53] Miller, G.A. (1947). Sensitivity to changes in the intensity of white noise and its relation to masking and loudness. J. Acoust. Soc. Am. 19: 609–619.

[54] Greenwood, D.D. (1993).The intensitive DL of tones: dependence of signal/masker ratio on tone level and on spectrum of added noise. Hear. Res. 65: 1–39.

Chapter 2

Classification of Hearing Loss

Waleed B. Alshuaib, Jasem M. Al-Kandari and Sonia M. Hasan

Additional information is available at the end of the chapter

http://dx.doi.org/10.5772/61835

Abstract

Hearing loss is the partial or total inability to hear sound in one or both ears. People with hearing loss make up a significant 5.3% of the world's population. The audiogram is an important tool used to determine the degree and type of hearing loss. This chapter presents hearing loss classification, which can aid in clinical diagnosis and help in finding appropriate therapeutic management. Hearing loss is classified based on ear anatomy, type of hearing loss, degree of the disease, and configuration of the audiogram. When the hearing loss is fully characterized, appropriate medical intervention can be assigned.

Keywords: Hearing loss, Audiometry, Conductive hearing loss, Sensorineural hearing loss

1. Introduction

Hearing is a very important sensation for human beings. It helps to understand the surrounding environment and can alert of any coming danger around us. Hearing is an essential means of communication. Hearing loss is the impairment of the ability to hear sound. The most quiet sounds that people can hear are between 25 and 40 decibel (dB). Anybody who suffers from mild hearing loss has difficulty keeping up with normal conversations. People who suffer from profound hearing loss are deaf and can hear nothing at all. Hearing loss can impact learning and development in children, including speech and language. In adults, hearing loss can greatly affect the overall quality of life, since it impacts social interaction and general well-being. Consequently, hearing loss can cause many difficulties in various aspects of life. Hearing loss can occur in different types and degrees of severity. In normal hearing, sound vibrations pass from the outer ear through the middle ear to the inner ear. In conductive hearing loss (CHL), vibrations cannot pass from the outer ear to the inner ear. In sensorineural hearing loss (SNHL), there is a dysfunction in the inner ear. In mixed hearing loss, there is a combination of conductive and sensorineural components. At the end of the inner ear (cochlea), thousands of auditory nerve fibers detect the high and low sound frequencies and transmit action potentials to the brain, which interprets the signal as sound. Repeated exposure to loud noise can damage the sound-sensitive hair cells in the inner ear, so it is important to protect hearing from harmful environments.

2. Hearing loss

2.1. Defining hearing loss, its prevalence, and incidence

Hearing loss, the most common form of human sensory deficit, is the partial or total inability to hear sound in one or both ears. It may be a **sudden** or a **progressive** impairment that gradually gets worse over time. Depending on the cause, it can be mild or severe, temporary or permanent. It may be a **bilateral** loss occurring in both ears or **unilateral**. Hearing loss may be **fluctuating**, that is, varying over time—improving at times and getting worse at other times. In other cases, hearing loss is **stable**, not changing at all with time. Hearing loss is caused by many factors, including genetics, age, exposure to noise, illness, chemicals, and physical trauma. Hearing loss may affect all ages, delaying speech and learning in children, and causing social and vocational problems for adults. According to the World Health Organization (WHO), there are 360 million persons in the world with hearing loss (5.3% of the world's population), and 32 million of whom are children [1]. The prevalence of hearing loss is increasing in adolescents and young adults and is associated with exposure to loud music. As for the aged, WHO reports that one-third of people above 65 years are living with disabling hearing loss [1]. Age-related hearing loss, **Presbycusis**, compromises the ability to discriminate sounds in environments with background noise. With the expected increase of 18–50% of the aging population in the coming years, the number of people with hearing loss will consequently grow [2]. Luckily, through early diagnosis and interventions, the majority of hearing loss cases are treatable. Understanding hearing loss and its classification is thus essential in improving the screening methods, preventive approaches, and in the management of the disease. A clear and concise description of the classification system for hearing loss based on the current state of scientific knowledge is important not only for clinical diagnosis and therapeutic management, but also for the use in medical research and education. In addition, a clear-cut explanation of the disease can aid patients who will themselves benefit from a better understanding of their hearing loss.

2.2. Understanding the audiogram

Hearing is examined by making the subject listen to a number of different pure tone signals through a pair of headphones or earplugs to record air conduction. An audiometer examines hearing ability by testing the threshold of hearing a sound signal at various frequencies (pitch, in cycles per second or Hz). Hearing threshold may be defined as how soft a sound may get before it becomes inaudible. Thresholds are measured in dB; the normal threshold is between 0 and 25 dB for adults and between 0 and 15 dB for children. Threshold is recorded on a graph known as the audiogram. The audiogram presents the sound frequency (ranging from low to high frequency) on the horizontal axis and sound intensity or loudness in dB on the vertical

http://dx.doi.org/10.5772/61835

axis. Right ear thresholds are recorded as red circles on the audiogram while the left ear thresholds are recorded as blue Xs. Figure 1 shows a typical audiogram with normal air conduction. A bone conduction test may be performed by bypassing the outer ear and the middle ear (also known as the air conductive pathway) to find the threshold when sound is delivered directly to the cochlea. This is done by placing a bone conductor, which sends tiny vibrations to the inner ear, on the mastoid process. A comparison between results from the air conduction test (that uses tone as stimulus) and the bone conduction test provides a better indication of whether hearing loss is due to conduction deafness or nerve deafness.

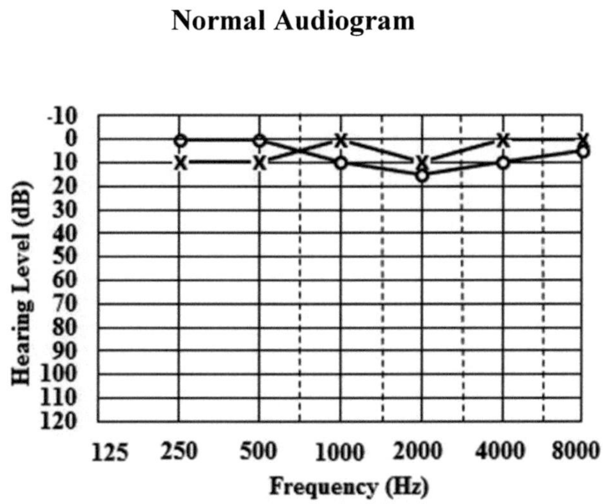

Figure 1. A typical audiogram with normal air conduction for both ears. Symbols: X, left ear air conduction; O, right ear air conduction.

2.3. Classifying hearing loss according to

2.3.1. Anatomy of the ear

An examination with attention to the anatomy of the ear is critical for establishing a hearing loss diagnosis. The auditory system is typically divided into three main sections: the outer, middle, and inner ears (Figure 2). **The outer ear** receives sound waves from the environment. The auricle captures sound and directs it into the external auditory canal (EAC) that ends at a thin diaphragm called the tympanum or ear drum. Obstruction of the EAC with ear wax or a foreign body, and inflammation of the canal, the auricle, or both (otitis externa) may produce hearing loss. Atresia, the congenital absence of the external ear canal and microtia, a congenital deformity where the pinna is underdeveloped, also cause hearing loss. Sound travels **the middle ear** as vibrations of three connected ossicles (malleus, incus, and stapes). Increase and decrease in sound-induced air pressure push and pull the tympanum, resulting in a mechanical response. The base of the first ossicle (the malleus) is attached to the tympanic membrane, while the last of the ossicles (the stapes) inserts in an opening called the oval window in the bony inner ear, the cochlea. The vibration of the incus drives the stapes deeper into the oval window and retracts it, pushing and pulling cyclically upon the liquid in the inner ear. The vibrating ossicles thus allow for the delivery of sound from the air-filled outer ear to the fluid-filled inner ear. Compromise of the middle ear's anatomy may lead to hearing loss. For example, bone growth in the ligamentous attachments of the ossicles can immobilize the ossicles and lead to severe deafness in a condition termed otosclerosis. Also of significance in the middle ear, attached to the stapes, is the stapedius muscle. This muscle contracts in response to loud sounds, thereby decreasing sound transmission to the inner ear and protecting it from acoustic insults. The cyclic motion created by the stapes displaces a liquid mass in **the inner ear**, which results in a traveling oscillating wave along the basilar membrane. The basilar membrane is elastic at the apex of the cochlea where it is most sensitive to low frequencies. On the other hand, the basilar membrane is stiff at the base of the cochlea and responds to high frequencies. Hair cells along the basilar membrane detect the frequency of the stimulus. The traveling wave pushes hair cells, depolarizing them and stimulating the afferent nerve fibers they are connected to, thereby transmitting the sound signal through the auditory (acoustic) nerve to the brain.

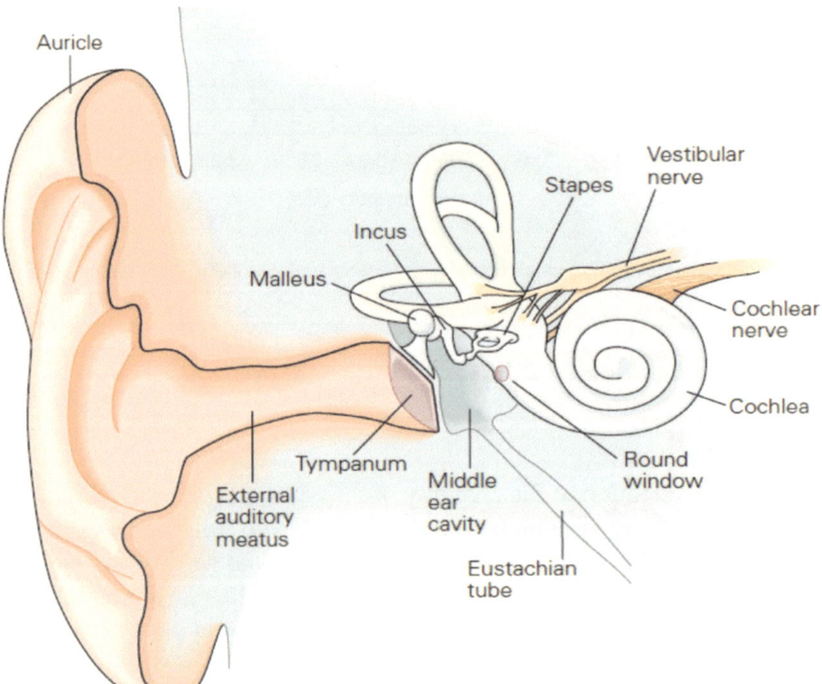

Figure 2. The structure of the human ear. The external ear, especially the prominent auricle, focuses sound into the external auditory meatus. Alternating increases and decreases in air pressure vibrate the tympanum. These vibrations are conveyed across the air-filled middle ear by three tiny, linked bones: the malleus, the incus, and the stapes. Vibration of the stapes stimulates the cochlea, the hearing organ of the inner ear. (Source [3]: Kandel et al. 2013 Principles of Neural Science. 5th ed.).

2.3.2. Type of hearing loss

Functionally, the human ear can be divided into two major divisions, the conductive division, associated with the areas responsible for air conduction (the outer ear and the middle ear) and the sensorineural division associated with the inner ear. Accordingly, the three main types of hearing loss are classified as conducive, sensorineural, and mixed hearing losses.

1. CHL is a type of hearing loss characterized by having better hearing thresholds for bone-conducted signals compared with air-conducted signals. CHL is usually associated with dysfunction located in the outer and/or middle ear while having a normal inner ear function. In CHL, the audiogram typically shows normal bone conduction (0–25 dB) and abnormal air conduction threshold levels (higher than 25 dB). According to the American Speech-Language-Hearing Association, a difference greater than 10 dB is considered a significant air–bone gap and requires the use of masking to eliminate a response from the ear not being tested, hence obtaining true thresholds from the test ear [4]. CHL can affect all frequency ranges. However, the low (250–500 Hz) or low and mid-range (250 Hz–2 kHz) frequencies are most commonly affected (Figure 3). The worst scenario of CHL is a loss of 60 dB or more. In the case of a total absence of the conductive function of the ear, sound waves can reach the cochlea through skull vibration and fluid movement. Most of the CHL cases are treatable with medication, surgery, amplification, assistive devices, or a combination of these. A common cause of CHL is the absence or malformation of the outer ear, ear canal, or middle ear structures. Atresia and microtia are such examples. Conductive pathologies include otosclerosis and cholesteotoma. The latter being a cystic mass of epithelial cells and cholesterol that occlude the middle ear and produce enzymes that may destroy adjacent bones. Tympanosclerosis, a consequence of chronic otitis media, is a condition of the middle ear cleft in which there are calcareous deposits in the tympanic membrane and the ossicular chain leading to CHL due to stiffness and reduced mobility. Other common causes of CHL include occlusion of the ear canal due to wax buildup or by a foreign object, perforated or scarred eardrum, outer ear (otitis externa) inflammation, or inner ear (otitis media) inflammation, trauma which causes injury to the tympanic membrane and/or ossicles, fluid accumulation, allergies, dysfunction of the Eustachian tube that normally drains fluid from the ear to the back of the throat, and benign tumors.

2. SNHL is a hearing loss that occurs as a result of damage in the cochlea or beyond, that is, either along the 8th cranial nerve or in the brain. SNHL can cause complete loss of hearing, despite the outer ear and middle ear being normal. Individuals with SNHL demonstrate similar air and bone conduction thresholds. The sensory component is usually due to the damage to the organ of Corti or to an inability of hair cells to stimulate the auditory nerve. The neural component refers to when damage is proximal to the cochlea and auditory nerve; the term retrocochlear damage is also used. SNHL may be the result of perinatal infections such as rubella, herpes, toxoplasmosis, syphilis, and cytomegalovirus. Birth complications associated with SNHL include asphyxia and low birth weight. Later onset causes of SNHL include infections such as meningitis, labyrinthitis, mumps, scarlet fever, and measles. Long exposure to loud noise induces SNHL by direct mechanical damage

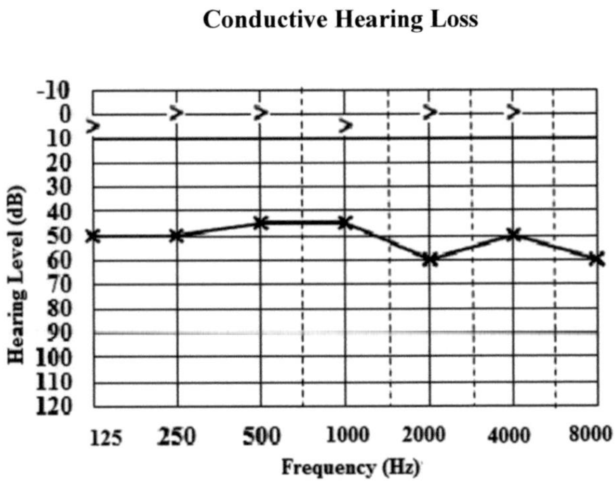

Figure 3. An audiogram with CHL for the left ear. The bone conduction is within normal range (0–25 dB) and the air conduction is in moderate—moderately severe range (moderate range: 41–55 dB, moderately severe:56–70 dB). Symbols: X, left ear air conduction; >, left ear bone conduction.

of inner ear structures. The US Occupational Safety and Health Administration require ear protection in the work area when an average exposure of 85 dB is reached. Severe SNHL may also occur after sudden exposure to a loud noise at 120–155 dB, for example from explosions, fireworks, gunfire, and music concerts. Other causes of SNHL include malformation of the inner ear, aging, Meniere's disease, drug-induced ototoxicity, and tumors such as acoustic neuroma. SNHL often cannot be reversed. Figure 4 shows an audiogram with SNHL.

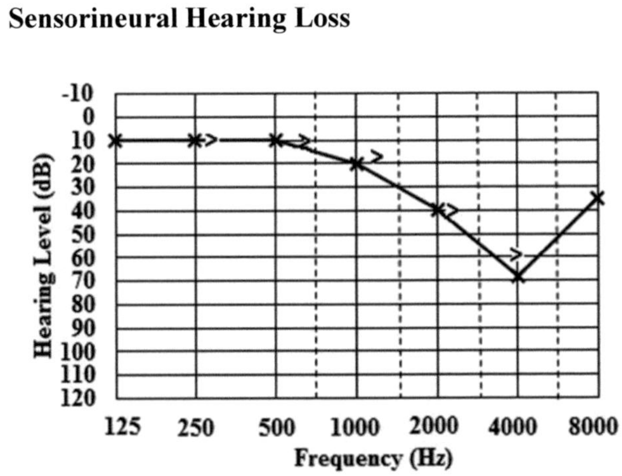

Figure 4. An audiogram with SNHL at high frequencies for the left ear. Both air conduction and bone conduction of high frequencies are in the mild (26–40 dB) to moderate range (41–55 dB) of hearing loss. Symbols: X, left ear air conduction; >, left ear bone conduction.

2. Mixed hearing loss is a type of hearing loss that has a combination of conductive and sensorineural damage in the same ear. Cases where both an air–bone gap greater than 10 dB and an elevated bone conduction threshold are observed suggest a mixed hearing loss. While the conductive component may be treated, the sensorineural component is more of a challenge. Figure 5 shows an audiogram with mixed hearing loss.

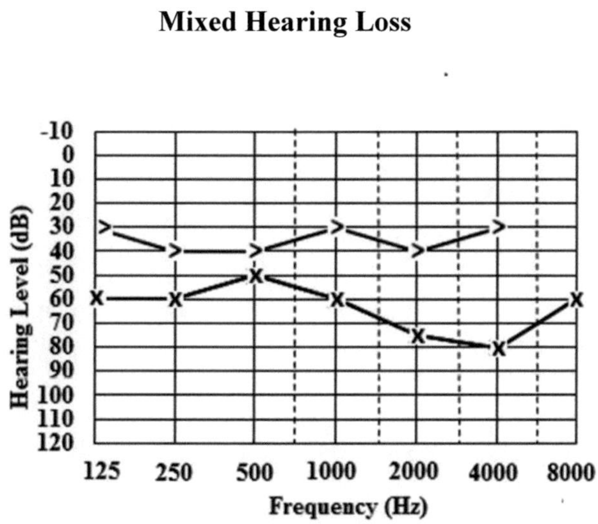

Figure 5. An audiogram with mixed hearing loss for the left ear. Both air conduction and bone conduction are in the abnormal range, with the air–bone gap generally greater than 10 dB. Symbols: X, left ear air conduction; >, left ear bone conduction.

2.3.3. *Degree of hearing loss*

Hearing loss can be classified according to the severity or degree of the disease. Hearing losses between 26 and 40 dB are considered mild, 41 and 55 dB moderate, 56 and 70 dB moderately severe, 71 and 90 dB severe, and greater than 91 dB profound (Table 1) [5, 6]. Severity of hearing loss is based on thresholds at individual frequencies. Once the type and degree of loss are established, an appropriate intervention may be assigned. This may include hearing aids, aural rehabilitation, cochlear implants, medical intervention, or surgery.

2.3.4. *Configuration of hearing loss*

Hearing losses may be categorized according to the audiometric configuration, that is, the shape or pattern of the audiogram across the frequency spectrum [7]. The configuration of an audiogram will tell you which sounds are best heard. A hearing loss that is more or less the same at all frequencies is depicted as a straight horizontal line on the audiogram and is thus appropriately called a **flat configuration**. In this configuration, thresholds across frequencies do not vary more than 20 dB from each other. In other words, a person with this type of loss needs the same amount of loudness to hear a sound regardless of the pitch. A person with a

Degree of hearing loss	Hearing threshold (dB HL)
Normal hearing	–10–15
Slight	16–25
Mild	26–40
Moderate	41–55
Moderately severe	56–70
Severe	71–90
Profound	>91

Table 1. Degree of hearing loss based on the hearing threshold. Source [5]: Clark JG: Uses and abuses of hearing loss classification. ASHA. 1981, 23:493–500.

sloping configuration has little or no hearing loss at low frequencies, severe loss at mid-frequency range, and profound loss at the higher frequencies. Ski-slope loss is another name for this configuration because the audiogram looks much like a ski slope with the top of the hill on the left and the slope dropping down to the right. Inversely, a **rising configuration** indicates that high-frequency sounds can be better heard than low-frequency sounds. This is a rare type of audiogram, an extreme example would be a person who is unable to hear thunder or explosive noise but can hear whispers across a room. Someone suffering from **cookie-bite or U-shaped configuration** hearing loss has one or more adjacent thresholds between 500 and 4,000 Hz ≥ 20 dB and so is likely to experience difficulty in hearing mid-frequency sounds, while maintaining the ability to hear high- and low-frequency sounds. Usually it is genetic; this type of hearing loss may progress over time. A **noise-notched configuration** indicates a hearing loss mostly between 3 and 6 kHz, while lower and higher frequencies are not affected. This configuration is observed in hearing loss due to noise exposure since sensory cells in the cochlea are more prone to noise damage in the 3-6 kHz frequency range than lower and higher frequencies. **High-frequency configuration** would show good hearing in the low frequencies and poor hearing in the high frequencies. Figure 6 shows the different configurations of hearing loss.

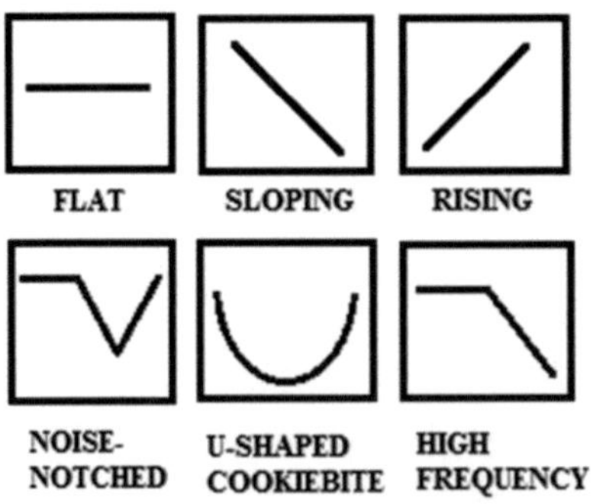

Figure 6. Hearing loss configurations.

http://dx.doi.org/10.5772/61835

Author details

Waleed B. Alshuaib[1*], Jasem M. Al-Kandari[2] and Sonia M. Hasan[3]

*Address all correspondence to: waleeds@hsc.edu.kw

1 Department of Physiology, Faculty of Medicine, Kuwait University, Kuwait

2 Audiology and Speech Clinic, Ahmadi Hospital, Kuwait

3 Department of Physiology, Faculty of Medicine, Kuwait University, Kuwait

References

[1] Multi-country assessment of national capacity to provide hearing care. WHO [Internet]. 2013. Available from: http://www.who.int/pbd/publications/WHOReportHearingCare_Englishweb.pdf [Accessed: 20150215].

[2] Millions of people in the world have hearing loss that can be treated or prevented—awareness is the key to prevention. WHO [Internet]. 2013. Available from: http://www.who.int/pbd/deafness/news/Millionslivewithhearingloss.pdf [Accessed: 20150215].

[3] Kandel et al. Principles of Neural Science. 5th ed. McGraw-Hill, New York; 2013; 655p.

[4] Guidelines for manual pure-tone threshold audiometry [Guidelines]. American Speech-Language-Hearing Association. 2005. Available from: www.asha.org/policy [Accessed: 20150215].

[5] Clark JG: Uses and abuses of hearing loss classification. ASHA. 1981 Jul;23(7):493–500.

[6] Baiduc RR, Poling GL, Hong O, Dhar S: Clinical measures of auditory function: the cochlea and beyond. Dis Mon. 2013 Apr;59(4):147–156. DOI: 10.1016/j.disamonth.2013.01.005.

[7] Pittman AL, Stelmachowicz PG: Hearing loss in children and adults: audiometric configuration, asymmetry, and progression. Ear Hear. 2003 Jun;24(3):198–205.

Chapter 3

Up to Date on Etiology and Epidemiology of Hearing Loss

Larissa Vilela Pereira and Fayez Bahmad Jr.

Additional information is available at the end of the chapter

http://dx.doi.org/10.5772/61845

Abstract

Deafness is one of the most common communication disorders in humans. Approximately one out of every thousand infants is born with a significant hearing deficit. The prevalence of hearing loss increases dramatically with age. By age 65 years, one out of three of us will suffer from hearing impairment sufficient to interfere with the understanding of speech. Hearing impairment is a very heterogeneous disorder with a wide range of causes. Worldwide, estimates from the World Health Organization are that hearing loss affects 538 million people. Hearing loss may be classified into three types: sensorineural, involving the inner ear, cochlea, or the auditory nerve; conductive, when the outer or middle ear structures fail to optimally capture, collect, or transmit sound to the cochlea; and mixed loss, which is a combination of conductive and sensorineural hearing loss. In this chapter, we propose to briefly define each cause of hearing loss as follows: (1) outer ear causes (congenital, infection, trauma, tumor, dermatologic, and cerumen), (2) middle ear causes (congenital, eustachian tube dysfunction, infection, tumors, otosclerosis, tympanic membrane perforation, middle ear barotrauma, and vascular), and (3) inner ear causes (congenital or hereditary, presbycusis, infection, Ménière disease, noise exposure, inner ear barotrauma, trauma, tumors, endocrine/systemic/metabolic, autoimmune hearing loss, Iatrogenic, ototoxic, and neurogenic).

Keywords: Etiology, hearing loss, conductive hearing loss, sensorineural hearing loss

1. Introduction

Deafness is one of the most common communication disorders in humans. Approximately one out of every thousand infants is born with a significant hearing deficit, and the prevalence of hearing loss increases dramatically with age. By age 65 years, one out of three of us will suffer from hearing impairment sufficient to interfere with the understanding of speech. Hearing impairment is a very heterogeneous disorder with a wide range of causes.[1]

Worldwide, estimates from the World Health Organization are that hearing loss affects 538 million people.[1]

Hearing loss may be classified into three types:

- Sensorineural: involving the inner ear, cochlea, or the auditory nerve
- Conductive: when the outer or middle ear structures fail to optimally capture, collect, or transmit sound to the cochlea
- Mixed loss: a combination of conductive and sensorineural hearing loss

2. Outer ear causes

The outer ear comprises the auricle and the external auditory canal (EAC), and all hearing loss related to the outer ear is by nature a conductive hearing loss.

2.1. Cerumen

Probably the most common cause of conductive hearing loss is the complete blockage of the EAC by a cerumen impaction. Some patients are not able to clear it on their own or use Q-tips that push the cerumen down the ear canal. These individuals may need periodic cleaning to enhance their auditory capabilities.

2.2. Infection

Infections may lead to blockage of the EAC due to the accumulation of debris, edema, or inflammation. Acute otitis externa usually develops as a result of local trauma coupled with contamination by bacteria (or occasionally fungi—otomycosis or viral—herpes zoster oticus) after swimming, showering, or exposure to hot and humid conditions. With complete obstruction, a conductive hearing loss results. Diabetes mellitus and other immunocompromised states can predispose to developing malignant otitis externa.[2]

2.3. Congenital

The auricle and the EAC are derived from different embryologic tissue, and each may develop without the full maturation of the other sites. The EAC develops from the 8th to the 28th week of gestation, and the auricle itself forms from remnants of the first and second branchial arch during the 12th and 20th weeks. Problems can occur anytime during this developmental phase, and it is possible to have a normal auricle but an atretic canal. The anatomical course of the facial nerve is frequently altered in malformations of the ear and temporal bone, but facial nerve function is rarely affected by the malformation. Conductive hearing losses that result from congenital malformations may range from mild to severe.

http://dx.doi.org/10.5772/61845

Malformation of the auricle is termed anotia when there is complete absence of an external ear and microtia when there is a vestige present. Anotia and microtia may cause mild to moderate conductive hearing loss.[2]

Congenital atresia of the EAC occurs in approximately 1 per 10,000 births and are usually associated with other craniofacial abnormalities such as Treacher–Collins syndrome, Pierre Robin syndrome, or Crouzon disease. The malformation occurs unilaterally 4 times more frequently than it does bilaterally (Figure 1).[3]

The severity of the atresia determines how well the child hears, and some patients with congenital atresia have associated inner-ear abnormalities, but these abnormalities typically do not cause sensorineural hearing loss. Atresia or significant stenosis of the EAC causes moderate to severe conductive hearing loss.[3]

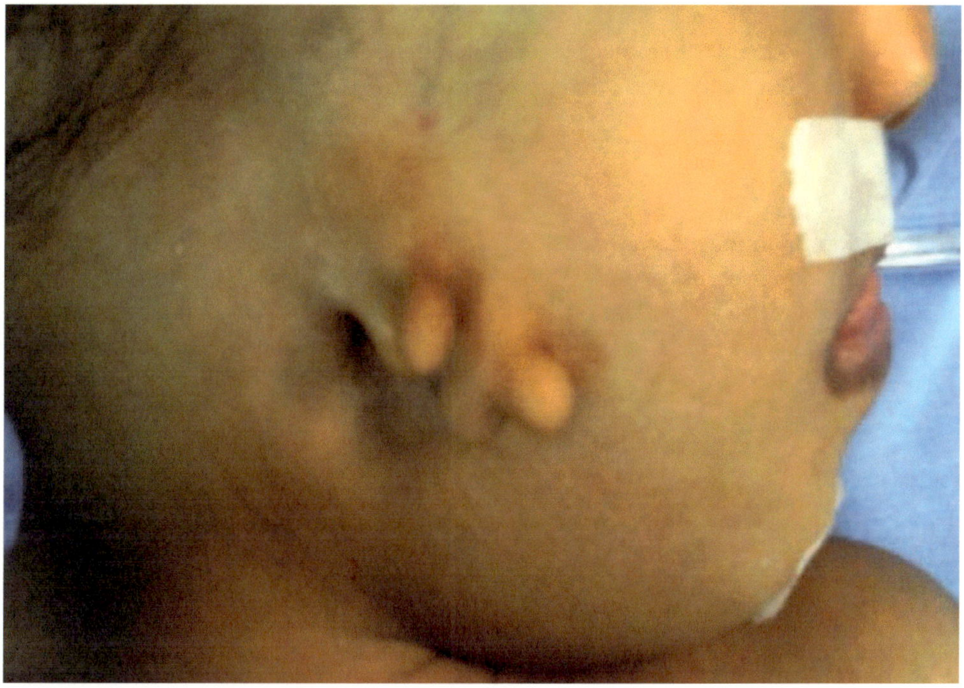

Figure 1. Congenital atresia of the EAC

2.4. Tumors

Malignant cancer of the ear canal is rare, and the most common histology type is squamous cell carcinoma. Other tumors include basal cell carcinoma, adenoid cystic carcinoma, adeno-carcinoma, and melanoma. Initially, cancer of the EAC is usually misdiagnosed as otitis externa because most patients complain of otorrhea, aural fullness, pain, itching, and hearing loss. However, after multiple failed attempts at treatment with ototopical drops and antibiotics, a biopsy of the EAC should be obtained. Treatment of these malignant tumors varies with the specific neoplasm.[4]

Benign bony growths may also occlude the EAC with a resulting conductive hearing loss. The two most common benign growths are exostosis and osteoma.

Exostosis are the most common solid tumor of the EAC. They are periosteal outgrowths that develop in the bony ear canal and occur mostly in men who have had repeated exposure to cold water. The lesions are often multiple, bilateral, and form in the suture lines of the EAC bones. Surgical removal is performed in cases of conductive hearing loss or recurrent otitis externa.[5]

Osteoma, in contrast, is a solitary bony growth that is most commonly attached to the tympanosquamous suture line. Similar to exostoses, osteomas are not treated until they become so large that they affect hearing by occlusion or repeated infections because debris cannot exit the EAC.[6]

Benign polyps may occur as a result of other otologic conditions, such as chronic ear infections or cholesteatoma. Occasionally, benign polyps can grow large enough to occlude the lumen of the external auditory canal.

2.5. Trauma

Penetrating trauma to the external auditory canal or meatus due to bullet, knife, or fracture may cause mild or profound conductive hearing loss, depending on the degree of EAC occlusion. Ototopical drops prevent otitis externa, and external auditory canal stenting is required initially to ensure that the EAC does not develop significant stenosis. Surgical intervention is reserved for cases of stenosis.

3. Middle ear causes

As with the outer ear, all hearing loss associated with the middle ear is conductive hearing loss.

3.1. Congenital malformation

Malformation of the ossicular chain can cause conductive hearing loss. The most common ossicular abnormality observed is a missing or malalignment of the crura of the stapes. However, it is usually an abnormal incus or malleoincudal joint that causes the conductive hearing loss. Computed tomography (CT) scan is virtually always needed in order to make this diagnosis, and in some cases, exploratory tympanostomy may be required.[2]

3.2. Eustachian tube dysfunction

The eustachian tube serves to provide normal middle ear pressure when opened and to protect the middle ear from reflux and nasopharyngeal bacteria when closed. Abnormal function occurs commonly in the setting of an upper respiratory infection (viral or bacterial), and it can also occur with allergies or tumors. It results in negative middle ear pressure causing reduction of tympanic membrane (TM) excursion and conductive hearing loss.

3.3. Infection

Acute otitis media (AOM) is a common childhood disorder that also frequently occurs in adults. Approximately 80% to 90% of all children will have developed at least one episode of OM by the time they enter school, and AOM accounts for more than 25% of the prescriptions for oral antibiotics annually.[7]

It is normally associated with pain, fever, and ear fullness as well as decreased hearing. Conductive hearing loss occurs because fluid filling the middle ear space prevents the TM from vibrating adequately, thereby diminishing movement of the ossicular chain.[8]

The middle ear may still be filled with serous or thick, tenacious fluid after the acute infection has been successfully treated. This fluid resolves within four to six weeks in 70% of cases. By an additional 12 weeks, 85% to 90% of all resolve the condition on their own. However, in the 10% to 15% in whom the fluid does not clear, it needs to be removed and the middle ear aerated in order to promote resolution of any conductive hearing loss. The fluid is usually cleared by either myringotomy and pressure equalization tube placement, or myringotomy and aspiration.[9]

3.4. Tympanic membrane perforation

Conductive hearing loss due to TM perforation is common. Clearly, the size, location, and nature of perforation will affect the degree of hearing loss. Small perforations and those located in the anterior–inferior quadrant cause the least amount of conductive hearing loss; near total or posterior–superior quadrant perforations have a much higher chance of causing significant hearing loss.[10]

Tympanic membrane perforations can arise as a consequence of either infection or trauma. Most perforations heal spontaneously. Occasionally, surgical correction is required, and repair of the perforation often corrects the conductive hearing loss.[7]

3.5. Otosclerosis

Otosclerosis is a primary disease of the temporal bone, leading to stapes ankylosis. Hearing loss is the main symptom. Complaints of continuous tinnitus and, eventually, vertigo are also observed. Otosclerosis is considered an autosomal dominant disease with incomplete penetrance being identified in three related genes: OTSC 1, OTSC 2, and OTSC 3. Treatment includes surgery, medical treatment, and sound amplification therapy alone or in combination.

3.6. Cholesteatoma

Cholesteatoma is a growth of desquamated, stratified, squamous epithelium within the middle ear space. Such collections of desquamated skin cells will erode bone slowly through a combination of pressure necrosis and enzymatic activity. Infection accelerates the process of bony destruction. The formation of a cholesteatoma typically occurs after a retraction pocket has formed in the posterior/superior quadrant, often the result of poor eustachian tube function. It may also occur after tympanic membrane trauma, such as a traumatic, inflammatory, or iatrogenic perforation, with implantation of squamous cells.[11]

Conductive hearing loss can occur as one or all ossicles become destroyed. Left untreated, cholesteatomas may erode the tegmen, the sigmoid sinus, or even the inner ear, resulting in labyrinthine fistula, which causes severe or profound sensorineural hearing loss and vertigo. Thus, untreated, they can cause lateral sinus thrombosis, sepsis, brain abscess, facial paralysis, and even death. Treatment is surgical, usually involving a mastoidectomy.[7]

3.7. Neoplasm

Malignant tumors such as Langerhans cell histiocytosis or squamous cell carcinoma may also occur in the middle ear and can cause conductive hearing loss. However, these entities are relatively rare when compared with cholesteatoma.

3.8. Middle ear barotrauma

Barotrauma occurs when a patient is exposed to a sudden, large change in ambient pressure, often during diving or flying. Middle ear pressure becomes more positive with respect to ambient pressure during ascent until the eustachian tube is forced open. On descent, ambient pressure exceeds middle ear pressure until swallowing opens the eustachian tube.

Pressure in the middle ear normally equilibrates with ambient pressure via the eustachian tube. However, if upon descent with flying or diving this equalization is prevented by mucosal edema secondary to an upper respiratory infection, pregnancy, or anatomic variations, the negative relative pressure in the middle ear can lead to its filling with serous fluid or blood or to inward rupture of the TM. Symptoms vary from a sensation of pressure to hearing loss and pain, which may suddenly be relieved with rupture of the TM.[12]

Overpressurization of the middle ear can occur during ascent with flying or diving, but TM rupture is rare.

3.9. Vascular

Glomus tumors are the most common benign neoplasm of the middle ear. They arise from paraganglionic tissue from the promontory of the middle ear or the adventitia of the dome of the jugular bulb and may rarely show malignant potential.[8]

As tympanic tumors grow, they tend to fill the middle ear, with resultant pulsatile tinnitus with or without conductive hearing loss. They also erode bone as they enlarge, especially inferiorly, causing damage to cranial nerves. In addition, tumors may impede upon the ossicular chain and TM, thereby decreasing motility of either or both structures.[2]

Treatment may include surgical resection, embolization, and radiation.

4. Inner ear causes

Disorders of the inner ear normally cause a sensorineural hearing loss. The etiology may be associated with the cochlea, eighth nerve, internal auditory canal, or brain.

4.1. Congenital or hereditary

Congenital hearing loss will be defined as any hearing loss that occurs at or shortly after birth that may be due to either a hereditary or nonhereditary cause. Nonhereditary etiologies involve an insult to the developing cochlea, including viral infections such as cytomegalovirus, hepatitis, rubella, toxoplasmosis, HIV, and syphilis. Some teratogenic medications may also affect the developing ear of the fetus, including recreational drugs, alcohol, quinine, and retinoic acid.[2]

Sensorineural hearing loss can be inherited in an autosomal dominant or recessive pattern; 90% is autosomal recessive, so that the children often have normal hearing parents. Sensorineural hearing loss also may be part of a syndrome or occur as a spontaneous mutation. The hearing deficit may be present at birth, be progressive from birth, or present when the child is older, or even early adult life. The most common testable genetic defect is an abnormal connexin 26.[1]

Congenital malformations of the inner ear also occur, these include anything from complete atresia to a common cavity of the cochlea. The most common malformation is a Mondini, where the normal two-and-one-half turns of the cochlea are replaced by one to one-and-one-half turns.

Patients who have congenital anomalies of either the inner or the middle ear may also develop perilymphatic fistulas (PLFs). PLFs alone can cause progressive or fluctuating sensorineural hearing loss.

4.2. Presbycusis

Presbycusis, or age-related hearing loss, is a common cause of hearing loss worldwide. This disorder is a complex and multifactorial, characterized by symmetrical progressive loss of hearing over many years. It usually affects the high frequencies of hearing, although its presentation and clinical course can be variable. Presbycusis has a tremendous impact on the quality of life of millions of older individuals and is increasingly prevalent as the population ages.[8]

Common complaints associated with presbycusis include the inability to hear or understand speech in a crowded or noisy environment, difficulty understanding consonants, and the inability to hear high pitched voices or noises. Tinnitus is often present.[2]

The prevalence of hearing loss increases with age, with up to 80% of functionally significant hearing loss occurring in older adults.

The World Health Organization (WHO) estimates that in 2025, there will be 1.2 billion people over 60 years of age worldwide, with more than 500 million individuals who will suffer significant impairment from presbycusis.

Hearing aids are able to benefit most patients with presbycusis, and cochlear implantation may benefit patients of any age who are not helped by hearing aids.

4.3. Infection

The most common infection of the inner ear is viral cochleitis in adults and meningitis in young children. Meningitis can access the cochlea by way of CSF-perilymph fluid connection and cause a profound sensorineural hearing loss by destroying the inner ear hair cells. Viral cochleitis usually manifests as a sudden sensorineural hearing loss and vertigo.[2]

Other causes of sudden sensorineural hearing loss include acoustic neuroma, perilymphatic fistula, Ménière disease, vascular insufficiency, multiple sclerosis, and other central etiologies. Although the primary etiology of sudden sensorineural hearing loss is almost always viral or a vascular ischemic event, patients with this presentation need to undergo audiometric evaluation as well as a magnetic resonance imaging (MRI) with gadolinium.

4.4. Ménière`s disease

Ménière`s disease is characterized by (1) spontaneous episodes of vertigo lasting several minutes to hours, (2) low-pitched tinnitus occurring or worsening during a vertiginous attack, (3) fluctuating low-frequency sensorineural hearing loss, and (4) aural fullness in the affected ear.[8]

The onset of symptoms is typically between the third and sixth decades, with a slight female preponderance. Endolymphatic hydrops is the main histopathologic correlate. Over time and with repeated attacks, the hearing deficit can become permanent and may even eventually involve all frequencies.

4.5. Noise exposure

Everyday noise exposure, compounded over time, has an impact upon our ability to hear. Constant exposure to loud noises can cause high-frequency sensorineural hearing loss, beginning with selective loss in 4000 Hz. With continued exposure, the notch widens and affects all high frequencies. Eventually, hearing loss can be seen in middle and lower frequencies. A short blast of loud noise also can cause severe to profound sensorineural hearing loss, pain, or hyperacusis. This usually involves exposure to noise greater than 120 to 155 dB.[2]

The mechanism by which excessive noise induces hearing loss includes direct mechanical damage of cochlear structures and metabolic overload due to overstimulation. Some potential metabolic effects are excess nitric oxide release that can damage hair cells, generation of oxygen free radicals that become toxic to membranes, and low magnesium concentrations that weaken hair cells by reducing the concentration of intracellular calcium.

http://dx.doi.org/10.5772/61845

Thus, hearing protection in the form of muffs or plugs is highly recommended anytime a person is exposed to loud noise.

4.6. Inner ear barotrauma

Barotrauma occurs when a patient is exposed to a sudden, large change in ambient pressure, often during diving or flying.

Inner ear barotrauma is a fairly uncommon injury but should be excluded in all cases of middle ear barotrauma. It can occur following the development of a sudden pressure differential between the inner and middle ear, leading to rupture of the round or oval window. The main symptoms are tinnitus, vertigo, and hearing loss. The resulting labyrinthine fistula and leakage of perilymph can result in permanent inner ear damage. The primary treatment of this complication is complete bed rest with head elevation to avoid increases in cerebrospinal fluid pressure. Deteriorating inner ear function generally requires tympanotomy and patching of the round or oval window.[2]

4.7. Trauma

Blunt trauma can result in sensorineural loss due to concussive forces of the inner ear fluids, which may cause a shearing affect on the cochlear organ of Corti. Blunt trauma may also lead to longitudinal or transverse temporal bone fracture.

The longitudinal type is most common (80%). It is usually caused by a blow to the temporal parietal region. Hearing loss is typically conductive and associated with tympanic membrane (TM) perforations and blood in the middle ear space.

A transverse fracture occurs following a blow to the occipital or frontal region (Figure 2). Fractures of this type usually run through the inner ear. If hearing is preserved to some degree, the most common reason for a conductive hearing loss is an ossicular injury, typically due to separation of the incudal stapedial joint and/or incus dislocation.[2]

Penetrating trauma typically causes sensorineural or mixed hearing loss. These injuries are usually due to gunshot wounds that upon impact cause significant temporal bone fractures.

4.8. Tumors

Most tumors of the inner ear are benign, although malignant tumors such as squamous cell carcinoma, sarcomas, adenoid carcinoma, and metastasis rarely occur. Benign bony tumors, including fibrous dysplasia and Paget disease, are also rare.[2]

The most common tumor that causes sensorineural hearing loss is an acoustic neuroma. Eighty percent of tumors arising in the cerebellopontine angle are acoustic neuroma. This is a benign tumor that usually arises from the Schwann's cells of the vestibular portion of the eighth cranial nerve. The most common complaint is an asymmetric progressive sensorineural hearing loss, which typically begins in the high frequencies and progresses to involve lower frequencies. Other symptoms include unilateral tinnitus, disequilibrium, dizziness, or headaches.[8]

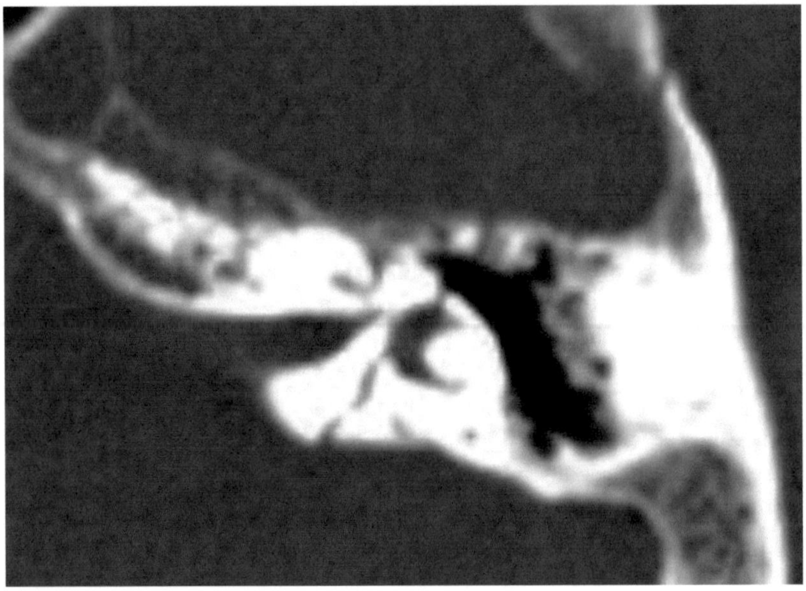

Figure 2. Transverse temporal bone fracture

4.9. Endocrine disorders

Various metabolic abnormalities have been known to either cause or be associated with sensorineural hearing loss. Thus, an evaluation of an unexplained sensorineural hearing loss should involve a complete laboratory evaluation to include the following: complete blood count with differential, blood sugar, thyroid function tests, and serologic test for syphilis.[2]

Diabetes has been associated with an approximately twofold increase in the prevalence of low- and midfrequency hearing impairment in adults; this might relate to the impact of diabetes on the vascular or neural components of the inner ear.[8]

Anemia or a white blood cell dyscrasia may lead to sensorineural hearing loss by an unknown mechanism that may involve decreased oxygenation, microblockage of vessels, or infection.

4.10. Autoimmune hearing loss

The autoimmune inner ear disease may be limited just to the ear, or it may be part of an overall systemic problem. Approximately one third of patients will have evidence of systemic autoimmune disorder such as Wegener granulomatosis, Cogan syndrome, rheumatoid arthritis, systemic lupus erythematosus, or polyarteritis nodosa.[2]

Autoimmune hearing loss is usually sensorineural, bilateral, and asymmetric, which is either fluctuating or progressive in nature.

The treatment choice for patients with autoimmune inner ear disease is high-dose glucocorticoids for up to 4 weeks. This often results in significant recovery of hearing.[2]

http://dx.doi.org/10.5772/61845

Cytotoxic medications such as cyclophosphamide, methotrexate, or azathioprine may be used if corticosteroids fail.

4.11. Ototoxicity

A great number of medications are known to cause damage to the ear. Anti-inflammatory, antibiotics, loop diuretics, antimalarials, chemotherapeutic agents, and ototopical medications may cause ototoxicity (Table 1).[8]

The hearing loss caused by antibiotic or chemotherapeutic agents usually begins at high frequencies, and with continued medication use, the hearing loss will become more pronounced and may even continue to worsen for a time after the drug is discontinued.

Several antibiotics cause ototoxicity. All oral aminoglycosides are ototoxic, and this effect is due to hair cell death from apoptosis. Different types of aminoglycosides show different patterns of ototoxicity. Streptomycin and gentamicin are primarily vestibulotoxic. Neomycin, amikacin, and tobramycin are primarily cochleotoxic.

Ototopical aminoglycoside drops have the potential to cause ototoxicity. However, it is believed that these medications do not have their normal ototoxic effect because the inflamed mucosa within the ear prevents significant drug penetration into the oval and round windows. Other oral antibiotics that can cause ototoxicity include erythromycin and tetracycline.

Medications		**Effects**
Antibiotics	**Aminoglycosides**	Vestibulotoxic
	Streptomycin	Vestibulotoxic
	Gentamicin	Cochleotoxic
	Neomycin	Cochleotoxic
	Amikacin	Vestibulotoxic and cochleotoxic
	Tobramycin	Cochleotoxic
	Macrolides	Cochleotoxic (synergism with aminoglycosides)
	Erythromycin	
	Glycopeptides	
	Vancomycin	
Anti-inflammatory	Aspirin (salicylates)	Cochleotoxic
Loop diuretics	Furosemide	Cochleotoxic (synergism with aminoglycosides)
Antimalarials	Quinine	Cochleotoxic
	Chloroquine	Cochleotoxic
Chemotherapeutic agents	Cisplatin	Cochleotoxic
Ototopical drops	Aminoglycoside drops (gentamicin and neomycin)	Potential ototoxicity in tympanic membrane perforation

Table 1. Medications related with ototoxicity

Many chemotherapeutic agents are known to cause hearing loss. These include cisplatin, 5-fluorouracil (5-FU), bleomycin, and nitrogen mustard. The worst ototoxicity occurs with cisplatin, which damage the outer hair cells of the basal turn of the cochlea, causing bilateral, symmetric, and high-frequency hearing loss.

High-dose aspirin (6–8 g/day) or other salicylates can cause a flat mild-to-moderate sensorineural hearing loss, but this is reversible with discontinuation of the drug.

Antimalarial medications such as quinine and chloroquine may also cause sensorineural hearing loss and tinnitus, but similar to salicylates, these effects are usually reversible. This is also true for high-dose nonsteroidal anti-inflammatory agents. Loop diuretics are an additional cause of temporary hearing loss and tinnitus.[2]

Heavy metals, including lead, mercury, cadmium, and arsenic, can all lead to hearing loss.

4.12. Neurogenic

Several neurologic disorders may cause sensorineural hearing loss: cerebrovascular accident or transient ischemic attack, Arnold–Chiari malformations (may stretch the auditory vestibular nerve, thereby causing hearing loss and/or vestibular complaints), and multiple sclerosis (can initially present as a sudden sensorineural hearing loss and/or vertigo). [2]

Author details

Larissa Vilela Pereira[1*] and Fayez Bahmad Jr.[2,3]

*Address all correspondence to: larissavilela24@yahoo.com.br

1 Otolaryngology Department, University of Sao Paulo School of Medicine, Sao Paulo, Brazil

2 Brasiliense Institute of Otolaryngology, Brasilia, Brazil

3 Health Science Faculty, University of Brasilia, Brasilia, Brazil

References

[1] Morton NE. Genetic epidemiology of hearing impairment. Ann N Y Acad Sci 1991;630:16–31.

[2] Cummings CW, Fredrickson JM, Harker LA, Krause CJ, Schuller DE. Otolaryngology Head and Neck Surgery. 2nd ed. 1993, Vol 4.

http://dx.doi.org/10.5772/61845

[3] Declau F, Cremers C, Van de Heyning P. Diagnosis and management strategies in congenital atresia of the external auditory canal. Study Group on Otological Malformations and Hearing Impairment. Br J Audiol 1999;33:313. (5)

[4] Gidley PW, Roberts DB, Sturgis EM. Squamous cell carcinoma of the temporal bone. Laryngoscope 2010;120:1144.

[5] DiBartolomeo JR. Exostoses of the external auditory canal. Ann Otol Rhinol Laryngol Suppl 1979;88:2.

[6] Hsiao SH, Liu TC. Osteoma of the external ear canal. Otol Neurotol 2003;24:960.

[7] Jung TTK, Hanson JB. Otitis media: surgical principles based on pathogenesis. Otolaryngol Clin North Am 1999;32:369–383

[8] Roeser RJ, Valente M, Hosford-Dunn H. Audiology. Diagnosis. 2nd ed. 2007

[9] Ryding M, Konradsson K, White P, Kalm O. Hearing loss after "refractory" secretory otitis media. Acta Otolaryngol 2005;125:250.

[10] Saliba I, Abela A, Arcand P. Tympanic membrane perforation: size, site and hearing evaluation. Int J Pediatr Otorhinolaryngol 2011;75:527.

[11] Sudhoff H, Tos M. Pathogenesis of attic cholesteatoma: clinical and immunohistochemical support for combination of retraction theory and proliferation theory. Am J Otol 2000;21:786.

[12] Farmer, JC Jr. Eustachian tube function and otologic barotrauma. Ann Otol Rhinol Laryngol 1985;120 suppl:45.

Chapter 4

Advances in Genetic Diagnosis and Treatment of Hearing Loss — A Thirst for Revolution

Sidheshwar Pandey and Mukeshwar Pandey

Additional information is available at the end of the chapter

http://dx.doi.org/10.5772/61218

Abstract

Despite the significant advances in understanding the molecular basis of hearing loss, precise identification of genetic cause still presents some difficulties, owing to phenotypical variation. Gene discovery efforts for hearing disorders are complicated by extreme heterogeneity. Mutations in some of these genes, such as *GJB2, MYO7A, CDH23, OTOF, SLC26A4, TMC1,* are quite common and responsible for hearing loss. Clinical exome sequencing is a highly complex molecular test that analyzes the exons or coding regions of thousands of genes simultaneously, using next-generation sequencing techniques. The development of a biological method for the repair, regeneration, and replacement of hair cells of the damaged cochlea has the potential to restore normal hearing. At present, gene therapy and stem cells are two promising therapeutic applications for hearing disorders. Gene therapy and stem cell treatment have still a long way to go before these treatments will be available to use in humans. Therefore, existing measures must focus on the prevention of hearing loss to decrease the frequency of genetic hearing loss. Over time, genetic diagnostic tests will become available most rapidly, followed by targeted gene therapy or various permutations of progenitor cell transplantation, and eventually, the preventive interventions for a wider range of hearing impaired patients.

Keywords: Genetic hearing loss, next generation sequencing, genetic evaluation, gene therapy, stem cell therapy

1. Introduction

Genetic hearing loss has diverse etiologies and approximately 1% of all human genes are involved in the hearing process [1]. It is estimated that at least two-thirds of cases of childhood-onset hearing loss have a genetic cause [2], with the remaining one-third caused by environmental factors, e.g., cytomegalovirus infection, meningitis, acquired conductive loss, and the impact of extracorporeal membrane oxygenation [3]. Many cases of later onset progressive hearing loss are genetic in origin, and genes also play an important role in progressive hearing loss associated with ageing. This chapter will deal with the ability to identify genetic problems or suspected genetic causes in hearing disorders, different types of gene mutation that causes deafness, genetic evaluation of hearing loss, special aspects of genetic tests such as next-generation sequencing, limitation of genetic testing, the development and evaluation of genetic treatment, management, prevention and genetic counseling, benefits of genetic research in deafness, and research needs/anticipating changes. It will conclude by the direction of possible future technological development in these aspects.

The majority of hearing loss is caused by mutations in the DNA (deoxyribonucleic acid) sequence of genes. There are four "bases" in a strand of DNA: adenine (A), guanine (G), thymine (T), and cytosine (C). The DNA also contains a monosaccharide sugar called deoxyribose and a phosphate group. According to base pairing rules (A with T, and C with G), hydrogen bonds bind bases of the two separate strands to make double-stranded DNA. Humans have approximately 30,000 genes. The DNA sequence of these genes provides the code for producing proteins (which consist of amino acids). The gene is located within a designated region on the chromosome and is composed of the different base pairs. The specific location on the chromosome where the gene is found is known as locus. For example, autosomal recessive deafness 1A (DFNB1A) is caused by mutation in the *GJB2* gene on chromosomal locus 13q11-q12. This means it is on the long arm of chromosome (q indicates the long arm) 13 somewhere in the range from band 1 of region 1 to band 2 of region 1 (11 or 12 represent the position on arm: 12- region 1, band 2). At times, changes (INDELs) occur in the DNA sequence of genes, such as a short segment of a gene is AGACATCATCTA and A has been replaced by a G at position 8 (AGACATCGTCTA) and C at position 4 has been deleted (AGAGATCGTTA), resulting in a mutation in the DNA sequence and affecting their functions such as a non-functioning protein may be produced or that protein may be missing altogether. If these mutations occur in a gene with important information for normal hearing, the result may be hearing loss, or in extreme cases, deafness.

2. Genetic causes of hearing loss

There are two types of hearing loss caused by genetics. About 30% of people with a genetic type of hearing loss are classified as syndromic, which involves other presenting abnormalities along with hearing impairment. Non-syndromic hearing loss occurs when there are no other problems associated with an individual other than hearing loss. From a genetic standpoint, this accounts for the other 70% of people, which attributes to the vast majority of genetic hearing loss.

The genetic basis is highly complex. There are many different ways that the DNA sequence of a gene can be changed, resulting in different types of mutation. The types of gene mutations include missence, nonsense, substitution, insertion, deletion, duplication, frameshifts, repeat expansion, splice site, and translocation. The chances of developing deafness caused by a mutated gene depend on whether the mutation is dominant or recessive. Dominant and recessive hearing loss results from the allelic mutation in some genes, syndromic and non-syndromic hearing loss is caused by mutations in the same gene, and recessive hearing loss may be caused by a combination of two mutations in different genes from the same functional group [4].

2.1. Non-syndromic hearing loss

The different gene loci for non-syndromic deafness are designated DFN (for DeaFNess). Based on the mode of inheritance, loci are named as A, B, X, and Y for autosomal dominant (DFNA), autosomal recessive (DFNB), X-linked (DFNX), and Y-linked (DFNY), respectively. The order in which the loci have been described is denoted by a number after these letters, e.g., DFNB1 is the first identified locus causing autosomal recessive HL [5, 6]. Earlier research reports that two-thirds of prelingual-onset sensorineural hearing loss (SNHL) is estimated to have a genetic etiology in developed countries, of which 70% is non-syndromic hearing loss (NSHL). However, 80% of NSHL is autosomal recessive non-syndromic hearing loss (ARNSHL), 20% is autosomal dominant (AD), and the remainder is composed of X-linked and mitochondrial forms [7-9]. NSHL demonstrates extreme genetic heterogeneity, with more than 55 autosomal dominant (deafness, neurosensory, DFNA), 80 autosomal recessive (deafness, neurosensory, DFNB), and 5 X-linked (deafness, neurosensory, DFNX) loci with 30, 55, and 4 causative genes, respectively, identified to date [10]. A fraction of these genes have been associated with both dominant and recessive HL. Furthermore, mitochondrial mutations can also underlie NSHL.

2.1.1. Autosomal dominant non-syndromic hearing loss

Autosomal dominant non-syndromic hearing loss (ADNSHL) is represented by heterogeneity of genetic and clinical features. ADNSHL is passed directly through generations. It is often possible to identify an autosomal dominant pattern through simple inspection of the family tree. Autosomal dominant traits usually affect males and females equally. ADNSHL associated with *GJB2* mutations is early-onset, moderate to severe, and (in contrast to autosomal recessive *GJB2* related deafness) typically progressive. Dominant *GJB2* mutations, however, often have pleiotropic effects. There is no frequent gene mutated in ADNSHL but *WFS1, KCNQ4, COCH,* and *GJB2* mutations are somewhat more frequent in comparison to the other reported genes [2, 11, 12]. Clinical manifestations and loci of known genes causing autosomal dominant non-syndromic hearing loss are summarized below in Table 1 [13, 14].

Locus Name	Gene	Onset/Decade	Audioprofile
DFNA1	*DIAPH1*	Postlingual/1st	Low frequency progressive
DFNA2	*KCNQ4*	Postlingual/2nd	High frequency progressive
DFNA2B	*GJB3*	Postlingual/4th	High frequency progressive
DFNA3	*GJB2*	Prelingual	High frequency progressive
DFNA3	*GJB6*	Prelingual	High frequency progressive

Locus Name	Gene	Onset/Decade	Audioprofile
DFNA4	*MYH14*	Postlingual	Flat/gently downsloping
DFNA5	*DFNA5*	Postlingual/1st	High frequency progressive
DFNA6/14/38	*WFS1*	Prelingual	Low frequency progressive
DFNA8/12	*TECTA*	Prelingual	Mid-frequency loss
DFNA9	*COCH*	Postlingual/2nd	High frequency progressive
DFNA10	*EYA4*	Postlingual/3rd, 4th	Flat/gently downsloping
DFNA11	*MYO7A*	Postlingual/1st	Flat/gently downsloping
DFNA13	*COL11A2*	Postlingual/2nd	Mid-frequency loss
DFNA15	*POU4F3*	Postlingual	High frequency progressive
DFNA17	*MYH9*	Postlingual	High frequency progressive
DFNA20/26	*ACTG1*	Postlingual	High frequency progressive
DFNA22	*MYO6*	Postlingual	High frequency progressive
DFNA23	*SIX1*	Prelingual	Downsloping
DFNA25	*SLC17A8*	Postlingual/2nd-6th decades	High frequency progressive
DFNA28	*GRHL2*	Postlingual	Flat/gently downsloping
DFNA36	*TMC1*	Postlingual	Flat/gently downsloping
DFNA39	*DSPP*	Postlingual	High frequency progressive
DFNA41	*P2RX2*	Postlingual	Flat progressive
DFNA44	*CCDC50*	Postlingual	Low to mild frequencies progressive
DFNA48	*MYO1A*	Postlingual	Progressive
DFNA50	*MIR96*	Postlingual/2nd	Flat progressive
DFNA51	*TJP2 & FAM189A2*	Postlingual/4th	High frequency progressive

Table 1. Clinical manifestations and locus of known genes causing ADNSHL. Adapted from [10, 14]

2.1.2. Autosomal recessive non-syndromic hearing loss

Autosomal recessive non-syndromic hearing loss at the *DFNB1* locus on chromosome 13q11-12 is characterized as congenital, typically non-progressive, mild to profound hearing impairment. The locus contains two genes, *GJB2* and *GJB6*. *GJB2* and *GJB6* are the most common mutated genes. *GJB2* is a small gene with a single coding exon. *GJB2* encodes connexin 26, a gap junction protein of the beta group with a molecular weight of 26 kd. The most common mutation is a deletion of a single guanine from a string of six *(35delG)*. This mutation accounts for more than two-thirds of identified mutations and results in a frame-shift with premature termination of the protein. Profound HL caused by *GJB2* gene mutations is found in 50% of the cases; 30% are severe, 20% moderate and 1-2% are mild cases [15]. *GJB2* mutation prevalence suggests that the overall prevalence of *GJB2* mutations is similar around the world, although specific mutations differ [16].

Mutations in the *GJB6* gene are the second most common genetic defect in hereditary hearing loss and lead to similar effects on abnormal expression of connexin protein Cx30. However, *GJB6* mutations are much less common than mutations in *GJB2*. In 1999, a research revealed the role for *GJB6*, i.e., adjacent to *GJB2* on chromosome 13, when a dominant mutation (T5M) was described [17]. The most common mutation in *GJB6*, however, is a >300-kb deletion that causes non-syndromic SNHL when homozygous, or when present on the opposite allele of a *GJB2* mutation [18]. *GJB6* is very similar to *GJB2* and only ~35 kb apart, but not interrupted by introns [4, 17]. Both genes are expressed in the cochlea where they can unite to form multi-unit hemichannels in the cell membrane, and function as an integral component of the potassium regulation in the inner ear. Clinical manifestations and locus of known genes implicated in autosomal recessive nonsyndromic hearing loss are summarized in Table 2 [10, 14].

Locus Name	Gene	Onset	Type
DFNB1	*GJB2*	Prelingual [1]	Usually stable
DFNB1	*GJB6*	Prelingual [1]	Usually stable
DFNB2	*MYO7A*	Prelingual, postlingual	Unspecified
DFNB3	*MYO15A*	Prelingual	Severe to profound; stable
DFNB4	*SLC26A4*	Prelingual, postlingual	Stable, progressive
DFNB6	*TMIE*	Prelinqual	Severe to profound; stable
DFNB7/11	*TMC1*	Prelinqual	Severe to profound; stable
DFNB8/10	*TMPRSS3*	Postlingual [2], prelingual	Progressive; stable
DFNB9	*OTOF*	Prelingual	Usually severe to profound; stable
DFNB12	*CDH23*	Prelingual	Severe to profound; stable
DFNB16	*STRC*	Prelingual	Severe to profound; stable
DFNB18	*USH1C*	Prelingual	Severe to profound; stable
DFNB21	*TECTA*	Prelingual	Severe to profound; stable
DFNB22	*OTOA*	Prelingual	Severe to profound; stable
DFNB23	*PCDH15*	Prelingual	Severe to profound; stable
DFNB24	*RDX*	Prelingual	Severe to profound; stable
DFNB25	*GRXCR1*	Prelingual	Moderate to profound; progressive
DFNB28	*TRIOBP*	Prelingual	Severe to profound; stable
DFNB29	*CLDN14*	Prelingual	Severe to profound; stable
DFNB30	*MYO3A*	Prelingual	Severe to profound; stable
DFNB31	*CHRN*	Prelingual	–
DFNB32/82	*GPSM2*	Prelingual	Severe to profound; stable
DFNB35	*ESRRB*	Unknown	Severe to profound
DFNB36	*ESPN*	Prelingual	–
DFNB37	*MYO6*	Prelingual	–

Locus Name	Gene	Onset	Type
DFNB39	*HGF*	Prelingual	Severe to profound; downsloping
DFNB49	*MARVELD2*	Prelingual	Moderate to profound; stable
DFNB53	*COL11A2*	Prelingual	Severe to profound; stable
DFNB59	*DFNB59*	Prelingual	Severe to profound; stable
DFNB61	*SLC26A5*	Prelingual	Severe to profound; stable
DFNB63	*LRTOMT*	Prelingual	Severe to profound; stable
DFNB67	*LHFPL5*	Prelingual	Severe to profound; stable
DFNB73	*BSND*	Prelingual	Severe to profound; stable
DFNB76	*SYNE4*	Prelingual	High frequency; progressive
DFNB77	*LOXHD1*	Postlingual	Moderate to profound; progressive
DFNB79	*TPRN*	Prelingual	Severe to profound; stable
DFNB84	*PTPRQ*	Prelingual	Moderate to profound; progressive

Table 2. Clinical manifestations and locus of known genes causing ARNSHL. Adapted from [10, 14].

2.1.3. X-Linked Non-Syndromic Hearing Loss

X-linked non-syndromic hearing loss is much rarer, accounting for 1-3% of hereditary deafness [19]. So far, there are only four genes that have been associated with X-linked non-syndromic hearing loss. These are: *PRPS1* on Xq22 that encodes phosphoribosyl pyrophosphate (PRPP) synthetase 1; *POU3F4* on Xq21, encoding a member of a transcription factor family that contains a POU domain; *SMPX* on Xp22 that encodes the small muscle protein; and *COL4A6* on Xq22 encoding the alpha-6 chain of type IV collagen. *COL4A6* is a protein-coding gene, type IV collagen having an important role in cochlea development. The *COL4A6* gene is located only ~500 kb away from the DFNX1/PRPS1 locus [20]. Clinical manifestations and locus of known genes causing X-linked nonsyndromic hearing impairment are summarized in Table 3 [10, 14].

Locus Name	Gene	Onset	Type and Degree	Frequencies
DFNX1 (DFN2)	*PRPS1*	Postlingual	Progressive sensorineural; severe to profound	All
DFNX2 (DFN3)	*POU3F4*	Prelingual	Progressive, mixed; variable, but progresses to profound	All
DFNX4 (DFN6)	*SMPX*	Postlingual	Progressive sensorineural; mild to profound	All
DFNX6	*COL4A6*	Postlingual	Progressive Sensorinueral, mixed; mild to severe	All

Table 3. Clinical manifestations and locus of known genes causing X-linked non-syndromic hearing loss. Modified from [10, 14].

2.1.4. Non-syndromic mitochondrial hearing loss

Mitochondrial DNA (mtDNA) mutations account for at least 5% of cases of postlingual, non-syndromic hearing impairment [21]. MtDNA mutations are classified as either large-scale rearrangements (partial deletions or duplications) that are usually sporadic or point mutations, which are usually maternally inherited, and concern genes responsible for protein synthesis (rRNAs or tRNAs), or genes encoding subunits of the electron transport chain (ETC) [22, 23]. Tang et al. reported that mitochondrial mutations by themselves are not sufficient to produce a deafness phenotype. Modifier factors such as nuclear and mitochondrial genes, or environmental factors such as exposure to aminoglycosides, appear to modulate the phenotypic manifestations [24].

The mutation most commonly associated with maternal inheritance is A1555G on gene *12S rRNA, MTRNR1* [25, 26]. Non-syndromic mitochondrial hearing loss is characterized by moderate-to-profound hearing loss and a pathogenic variant in either *MTRNR1* or *MTTS1*. Pathogenic variants in *MTRNR1* can be associated with the predisposition to aminoglycoside ototoxicity and/or late-onset sensorineural hearing loss. [27].

The use of streptomycin, and to a lesser extent other aminoglycoside antibiotics, can cause hearing loss in genetically susceptible individuals. These drugs are known to exert their antibacterial effects at the level of the decoding site of the small ribosomal subunit, causing miscoding or premature termination of protein synthesis [28-30]. The hearing loss is primarily high frequency and may be unilateral. Mitochondrial non-syndromic sensory neural hearing loss (SNHL) is also associated with the A7445G, 7472insC, T7510C, and T7511C mutations in the tRNASer (UCN) gene,*MTTS1* [30, 31]. Mitochondrially inherited non-syndromic hearing loss can be caused by mutation in any one of several mitochondrial genes, including *MTRNR1, MTTS1, MTCO1, MTTH, MTND1,* and *MTTI* (Table 4).

Gene	Mutation	Possible additional symptoms
MTRNR1 (12S rRNA)	1555A->G	Aminoglycoside induced/worsened
	1494C->T	Aminoglycoside induced/worsened
	961(mutations)	Aminoglycoside induced/worsened
	827A>G	Aminoglycoside induced
MTTS1 (tRNASer(UCN))	7445A->G	Palmoplantar keratoderma
	7472insC	Neurological dysfunction, including ataxia, dysarthria, and myoclonus
	7510T->C	No additional symptoms
	7511T->C	No additional symptoms
MTCO1	7444G>A	Aminoglycoside associated; associated with *MTRNR1* 1555A >G
MTTH	12201T-C	No additional symptoms
MTND1	3388C-A	Tinnitus and BPPV associated
MTTI	4295A-G	Hypertrophic cardiomyopathy

Table 4. Identified mitochondrial DNA mutations in hearing loss. Modified from [10].

2.2. Syndromic hearing loss

Syndromic forms of hearing loss are less common than non-syndromic forms. To date, more than 400 genes responsible for syndromic hearing loss have been identified [32]. These can include syndromes transmitted in Mendelian or monogenic, syndromes due to chromosomal anomalies, syndromes due to multi-factorial influences, or syndromes due to a combination of these. Syndromic hearing loss can be conductive, sensorineural, or mixed.

Many of the syndromes associated with SNHL do not usually demonstrate gross inner ear anomalies. However, inner ear malformations are common in numerous syndromes. In some cases, the existence of specific inner ear anomalies may be characteristic of certain syndromes such as in BOR syndrome, Waardenburg syndrome, or X-linked deafness with stapes gusher or CHARGE syndrome. SNHL presenting later in life is often related to inner ear infections or inflammatory conditions, trauma, or tumor [33].

Mutations in the same gene may cause syndromic hearing loss in one individual and non-syndromic hearing loss in another. The most common autosomal dominant form is Waardenburg syndrome. The most common autosomal recessive forms are Pendred syndrome and Usher syndrome. Syndromic hearing loss may be transmitted as an autosomal recessive, autosomal dominant, X-linked, or matrilineal trait. Some of the genetics forms of syndromic hearing loss and their main clinical features are given in Table 5 [34].

Syndrome	Main Clinical Features	Genetics	Hearing loss
Waardenburg syndrome (AD)*	· Type 1: dystopia canthorum, iris heterochromy, brilliant blue eyes, broad nasal root, premature, graying of hair, white forelock, and vestibular dysfunction	*PAX3*	Sensorineural hearing loss
	· Type 2: similar phenotype except dystopia canthorum	MITF, SNAI2	
	· Type 3 (Klein-Waardenburg syndrome): upper extremity abnormalities other Type 1 clinical features	*PAX3*	
	· Type 4 (Waardenburg-Shah syndrome): pigmentation abnormalities and Hirschsprung's disease other Type 2 clinical features	*EDN3*, *SOX10* and *EDNRB*	
Charge syndrome (AD)	· Choanal atresia · Coloboma · Characteristic ears · Cranial nerve anomalie · Cardiovascular malformations	Mutations in *CHD7* are detected in more than 75% of CHARGE	Severe-to-profound asymmetrical mixed losses

Syndrome	Main Clinical Features	Genetics	Hearing loss
	· Genital hypoplasia · Cleft lip/palate · Tracheoesophageal fistula · Growth deficiency · Developmental delay	patients SEMA3E	
Pierre Robin Sequence (AD)	· Micrognathia · Glossoptosis · Cleft palate	Genetic heterogeneity	Typically conductive and bilateral
Stickler syndrome (AD)	· Long and flat face · Malar and mandibular hypoplasia · Small nose with a depressed nasal bridge and anteverted nares · Altered vision · Joint problems	Mutations in *COL2A1*, *COL9A1*, COL9A2, *COL11A1*, and *COL11A2* genes	Both sensorineural and conductive
Branchio-oto-renal (BOR) syndrome (AD)	· Branchial cleft, cysts, or fistulae · Ear abnormalities · Kidney abnormalities	*EYA1*, *SIX1*, and *SIX5* mutations	Sensorineural, conductive, or mixed hearing loss
Treacher- Collins syndrome (AD)	· Zygomatic arches hypoplasia · Hypoplasia of supraorbital rims · Micrognathia · Narrow face · Antimongoloid slant of the eyes and hypertelorism · Coloboma of the lower lid with deficiency of cilia medial to the coloboma · Large nose is with hypoplastic alae · Down-turning mouth · Cleft palate · External ear abnormalities	Genetic heterogeneity: TCS-1, TCS-2 and TCS- 3 have been related to mutations in *TCOF-1*, *POLR1D* and *POLR1C* respectively	About 40-50% of patients with Treacher Collins have conductive hearing loss. Few cases of mixed hearing loss have been described.
Apert syndrome (AD)	· Craniosynostosis · Frontal bossing · Wide set eyes	*FGFR2* mutations	Mild to moderate conductive hearing loss

Syndrome	Main Clinical Features	Genetics	Hearing loss
	· Hypoplastic midface · Proptosis · Small upper jaw · Syndactyly		
Crouzon syndrome (AD)	· Synostosis · High forehead · Proptosis · External strabismus · Hypertelorism · Prognathism · Hypoplastic upper jaw	*FGFR2*	Conductive hearing loss
Saethre- Chotzen syndrome (AD)	· Brachycephaly · Low frontal hair line · Flattened nasofrontal angle · Widely spaced eyes · Ptosis · Facial asymmetry · Syndactyly · Broad or duplicated thumb or hallux	*TWIST1*	Conductive or mixed
Pfeiffer syndrome (AD)	· Broad face is midface hypoplasia · Prognatism · High forehead, flat occiput, hypertelorism · Swallowing orbits which cause proptosis · Skull malformation · Limb abnormalities	*FGFR1* & *FGFR2*	Conductive
Townes-Brock syndrome (AD)	· Anus imperforatus · Rectovaginal · Rectoperineal fistula · External ear anomalies · Thumbs malformation	It is caused by mutations in *SALL1*	Sensorineural or conductive hearing loss
Miller syndrome (AR** or AD)	· Malar hypoplasia · Micrognathia · Down-slanting eyes	*DHODH*	Conductive hearing loss- mainly due to

http://dx.doi.org/10.5772/61218

Syndrome	Main Clinical Features	Genetics	Hearing loss
	· Coloboma · Cleft palate · Limb defects		anomalies of middle ear
Nager syndrome (Sporadic, AD or AR)	· Limbs abnormalities · Maxillar hypoplasia · Micrognatia	Not known	Conductive or mixed hearing Loss
Goldenhar syndrome (Sporadic, AR or AD)	· Hemifacial microsomia · Auricular malformations · Vertebrae abnormalities · Facial cleft · Ocular abnormalities · Congenital heart diseases	Genetic heterogeneity	Ranges from mild to moderate conductive impairment and severe to profound sensorineural hearing loss
Usher Syndrome (AR)	· Type 1: vestibular dysfunction onset of retinitis pigmentosa in childhood	*MYO7A, USH1C, CDH23, PCDH15,USH1G* & *CIB2,*	Profound hearing Loss
	· Type 2: normal vestibular response retinitis pigmentosa begins in the second decade of life	*VLGR1, WHRN, PDZD7*	Mild to moderate hearing loss
	· Type 3: variable vestibular response, variable onset of retinitis pigmentosa	*USH3A, CLRN1*	Progressive hearing loss
Pendred syndrome (AR)	· Abnormal iodine metabolism (goiter)	*SLC26A4* , *FOXI1,* KCNJ10	Usually bilateral, severe to profound
Jervell & Lange-Nielsen (AR)	· SIDS, syncopal episodes prolongation of the QT interval	KCNQ1, KCNE1	Sensorineural hearing loss
Perrault syndrome (AR)	· Ovarian dysfunction in females, · Intellectual disability, · Loss of sensation and weakness in the limbs	HSD17B4, HARS2, LARS2	Sensorineural hearing loss
Alport syndrome (AR,AD, X-Linked)	· Renal abnormalities including glomerulonephritis, hematuria, and renal failure	COL4A3, COL4A4 and COL4A5	Progressive sensorineural hearing loss

Syndrome	Main Clinical Features	Genetics	Hearing loss
	· Hearing loss usually begins in the adolescent years		
Mohr-Tranebjaerg syndrome (X-Linked)	· Visual disability · Dystonia, fractures · Intellectual disability	*TIMM8A*	Progressive hearing loss
Norrie Syndrome (X-Linked)	· Eye disorder · Developmental delays in motor skills · Mild to moderate intellectual disability	NDP	Sensorineural Progressive HL

*AD- Autosomal dominant inheritance, **AR- Autosomal recessive inheritance

Table 5. Syndromic hearing loss and their clinical features. Modified from [34].

3. Genetic evaluation of hearing loss

Despite the significant advances in understanding the molecular basis of hearing loss, precise identification of genetic cause still presents some difficulties due to phenotypical variation. Gene discovery efforts for hearing disorders are complicated by the extreme heterogeneity. Usher syndrome or Jervell and Lange-Nielsen syndrome, which can be mistaken for nonsyndromic hearing loss, where Usher syndrome can be caused by mutations in several different genes. We must therefore have a clear understanding of the different types of diagnostic tests available to patients, including karyotyping, RFLP, FISH, microarray, clinical exome sequencing, preimplantation genetic diagnosis, and newborn genetic screening. Establishing a genetic diagnosis of hearing loss is a critical component of the clinical evaluation of hearing impaired persons and their families. If a genetic cause of hearing loss is determined, it is possible to provide families with prognostic information, recurrence risks, and improved habilitation options [9].

The identification of genes or genetic cause for hearing loss is a breakthrough approach. First we have to rule out non-genetic causes, then syndromic causes, and then look for non-syndromic causes. Mutations in some of these genes, such as *GJB2, MYO7A, CDH23, OTOF, SLC26A4, TMC1* are quite common for responsible of hearing loss. *GJB2* mutations are the most frequent cause of autosomal recessive non-syndromic hearing loss (ARNSHL) and account for about 20% of the cases, therefore routine screening begins with *GJB2* analysis [35]. Newborns that are diagnosed with severe-to-profound HL (in the absence of other abnormal findings on physical examination) are analyzed for mutations in the *GJB2* gene. For abnormalities such as an enlarged vestibular aqueduct indicated by imaging of the inner ear, the *SLC26A4* gene is analyzed. It is exceptional to find any gene other than *GJB2* and *SLC26A4* that is routinely analyzed in DNA diagnostics. In such cases, a positive result is only obtained in less than 20% of deaf children for which DNA diagnostics is requested [2, 36]. The key challenge lies in determining which gene is responsible in a patient with hearing loss. Sequencing all genes by traditional DNA sequencing technology is labor-intensive and not cost-effective [35, 36]. In such case, next-generation sequencing offers rapid sequencing of the entire human genome compared to traditional molecular testing that focuses on a single gene at a time. However, Sanger sequencing is still recommended for first-line diagnostics. It is currently the standard for molecular diagnosis of unknown point mutations in known genes. Screening can be cost-effective in individuals with genetically heterogeneous hearing loss phenotypes when a single gene is responsible for a significant percentage of cases.

3.1. Next-generation sequencing

With the fast development and wide applications of next-generation sequencing (NGS) technologies, genomic sequence information is within reach to aid the achievement of goals to decode life mysteries and improve life qualities. Today, NGS-based tests are rapidly replacing traditional tests, which include many single gene-sequencing tests for hearing loss. These tests use disease-targeted exon capture, whole-exome sequencing (WES), or whole-genome sequencing (WGS) strategies. The main advantage of these tests is that they address the problem of genetic heterogeneity, where many different genes result in phenotypes that cannot be easily distinguished clinically [36-39]. NGS also offers sequencing of very large gene or in presence of substantial locus heterogeneity, where it may be difficult to analyze the same gene by comprehensive Sanger sequencing.

NGS systems are typically represented by SOLiD/Ion Torrent PGM from Life Technologies, Genome Analyzer/HiSeq/MiSeq/NextSeq from Illumina, and GS FLX Titanium/GS Junior from Roche. Today, Illumina dominates the genome sequencing market, where instrument versatility, high throughput and accuracy, turnaround speed, faster and simpler sample preparation, and supportive data analysis software make it a driving force and the clear winner as of now. Their technology creates new applications and also decipher many existing genetic research and clinical diagnostic markets.

Targeted genomic capture and massively parallel sequencing technologies are revolutionizing genomics by making it possible to sequence complete genomes of model organisms. However, the cost and capacity required are still high, especially considering that the functional significance of intronic and intergenic noncoding DNA sequences is still largely unknown. One application that these technologies are well suited for is the re-sequencing of many selected parts of a genome, such as all exons, from a large set of genes. This requires that the targeted parts of the genome are highly enriched in the sample. Recent technological changes, such as genome capture, genome enrichment, and genome partitioning, have successfully been used to enrich large parts of the genome [40-42]. The targeted fragments can subsequently be captured using solid- or liquid-phase hybridization assays [43, 44].

Clinical exome sequencing or whole-exome sequencing is a highly complex molecular test that analyzes the exons or coding regions of thousands of genes simultaneously from a small sample of blood, using NGS techniques. Exome sequencing is especially valuable when a patient's symptoms suggest numerous possible genetic causes. The whole-exome sequencing test sequences base by base with the required depth of coverage to achieve accurate consensus sequence rather than limiting the testing to a single gene or panel of genes and incurring diagnostic delays and escalating costs. It is possible to identify point mutations, insertions, deletions, inversions, and rearrange the exome.

Hearing status	Locus/disorder	Gene	Strategy	References
Nonsyndromic Recessive	DFNB79	*TPRN*	Targeted enrichment of genomic locus	[48]
	DFNB82	*GPSM2*	Whole exome	[49]
	DFNB84	*OTOGL*	Whole exome	[50]
Dominant	DFNA4	*CEACAM16*	Whole exome	[51]
	DFNA41	*P2RX2*	Targeted enrichment of genomic locus	[52]
X-Linked	DFNX4	SMPX	Targeted enrichment of genomic locus	[53]
Syndromic	Perrault syndrome	*HSD17B4*	Whole exome	[54]
	Perrault syndrome	*HARS2*	Targeted enrichment of genomic locus	[55]
	Carnevale, Malpuech, Michels, and oculo-skeletal-abdominal syndromes	*MASP1*	Whole exome	[56]
	Hereditary sensory and autonomic neuropathy type 1 (HSAN1) with dementia and hearing loss	*DNMT1*	Whole exome	[57]

Table 6. Deafness genes identified using genomic capture and massively parallel sequencing.

Among NGS applications, whole-exome sequencing is a cost-effective alternative to whole-genome sequencing. The total size of the human exome is ~30 Mb, which comprises ~180,000 exons that are arranged in about 22,000 genes and constitute about 2-3% of the entire human genome, but contains ~85% of known disease-causing variants. The exome refers to the portion of the human genome that contains functionally important sequences of DNA that direct the body to make proteins essential for the body to function properly. Research revealed that most of the errors that occur in DNA sequences are usually located in the exons that lead to genetic disorders. Consequently, sequencing human exome is considered to be an efficient method to discover the genetic cause of hearing disorders. Currently, sequencing whole genomes is still a substantial undertaking, which is not a routine procedure that can be done on hundreds of samples. At present, exome sequencing represents an alternative in which, approximately 30-70 Mb sequences encompassing exons and splice sites are targeted, enriched, and sequenced using commercially available sequence capture methods. Several Human Exome Sequence

Capture kits are now commercially available. These include the Agilent SureSelect Human All Exon Kit, the Illumina Nextera Rapid Capture Exome and Nextera Rapid Capture Expanded Exome Kit, the TargetSeq In-solution Target Enrichment Kit from Life Tech/Applied Biosystems, and SeqCap EZ Exome from Roche NimbleGen. Clinical exome sequencing should be considered in the diagnostic assessment of a phenotype individual when a genetic disorder is suspected clinically, but limited genetic testing is available clinically, the patient's features are unclear or atypical, there are multiple genetic conditions as part of the differential diagnosis, and a novel or candidate gene is suspected but has yet to be discovered.

Hundreds of syndromic forms of deafness have been described, and for many of them, the underlying genes still await discovery. Since the introduction of the first NGS technology in 2004, more than 1,000 NGS-related manuscripts have been published. Until now, approximately a dozen of genes for HL have been successfully determined using NGS [45-47] (Table 6).

3.1.1. Sequencing panels

Consider a case where there is an interest in a large but limited subset of particular genes, not the whole genome, or even the whole exome, but more than just one or two genes. This sort of situation frequently arises in the context of oncology, where the characterization of a set of oncogenes on a set of pathways can help stratify cases and select the best therapeutic options. These may consist of 30-150 particular target genes, with a desire to have high throughput by analyzing multiple different specimens within a single NGS run. Generally referred to as "NGS panels," this is a third form of library which, depending on design, may start with extracting genomic DNA from a test sample where selection of targets of interest is performed. This can be by gene-specific PCR, leading to a pool of amplicons (already of the desired length, although in this case with defined endpoints), by hybridization capture, or by selective genomic DNA coding only for particular genes. This genetic material is then a very focused subset of the source genome from which to prepare the library material for dispersion and sequencing, following either of the paths above as appropriate to the sample type (note that for a direct PCR amplified genomic DNA panel type, the size shearing and adapter ligation steps may be dispensed with as these are effectively carried out in the PCR step).

A particularly clever aspect of NGS panels is that it is possible, either in the direct PCR stage for genomic DNA-based panels or in the adapter ligation step for exome-based panels, to use PCR primers or adapters, respectively, which contain an internal sequence element (commonly referred to as a "barcode") that is distinct to each sample prepared. This then allows multiple panel libraries from different samples to be mixed together prior to the dispersion and actual sequencing steps. By doing this, each individual sequence read will start with a sample-unique "barcode," allowing it to be associated back to the sample of origin. This allows many different unrelated panel sample libraries to be mixed together in one dispersion and sequencing run, thereby taking full advantage of the massively parallel nature of NGS technology and allowing for high throughput with respect to the number of samples per run. This makes panels highly cost-effective and of relatively low labor input on a per-sample basis. Depending on the type of research or clinical question being addressed in an NGS assay, the choice of the best method helps to make results cost-effective and most directly meaningful.

Different panels designed to diagnose hearing loss include:

- Hearing Loss Panel Tier 1—testing for mutations in *GJB2, GJB6, MTRNR1*, and *MTTS1* that account for 40% of the genetic causes of hearing loss. Reflex testing to OtoSeq® Hearing Loss Panel is an option for patients with normal Tier 1 results. This panel contains 23 genes, which identifies an estimated 80% of the genetic causes of hearing loss.
- OtoGenomeTM Test Panel offered by Partners Healthcare. This test panel simultaneously screens 87 genes known to cause both non-syndromic hearing loss and syndromes that can present as isolated hearing loss, such as Usher, Pendred, Jervell and Lange-Nielsen (JLNS), Branchio-Oto-Renal (BOR), Deafness and Male Infertility (DIS), Perrault, and Waardenburg syndromes.

3.1.2. NGS data analysis

The large amount of data derived from NGS platforms imposes increasing demands on statistical methods and bioinformatic tools for the analysis. Although the NGS platforms rely on different principles and differ in how the array is made, their work flows are conceptually very similar. All of them generate millions or billions of short sequencing reads simultaneously. Several layers of analysis are necessary to convert these raw sequence data into understanding of functional biology. These include alignment of sequence reads to a reference, base-calling and/or polymorphism detection, de novo assembly from paired or unpaired reads, and structural variant detection (Figure 1). To date, a variety of software tools are available for analyzing NGS data. Although tremendous progress has been achieved over the last several years in the development of computational methods for the analysis of high-throughput sequencing data, there are still many algorithmic and informatics challenges remaining. For example, even if a plethora of alignment tools have been adapted or developed for the reconstruction of full human genotypes from short reads, this task remains an extremely challenging problem. Also, when a high-throughput technology is used to sequence an individual (the donor), any genetic difference between the sequenced genomes and a reference human genome—typically the genome maintained at NCBI—is called the variant. Although this reference genome was built as a mosaic of several individuals, it is haploid, and may not contain a number of genomic segments present in other individuals. By simply mapping reads to the reference genome, it is impossible to identify these segments. Thus, de novo assembly procedures should be used instead. Nonetheless, NGS technologies continue to change the landscape of human genetics. The resulting information has both enhanced our knowledge and expanded the impact of the genome on biomedical research, medical diagnostics, and treatment, and has accelerated the pace of gene discovery [47].

Clinical diagnostic using NGS technologies may be applicable in such cases where clinicians consider a non-syndromic hearing disorder, especially after negative results on tests for mutations in the autosomal recessive *DFNB1* locus for *GJB2* or *GJB6*, according to recently published guidelines [39, 58]. Updated guidelines from the American College of Medical Genetics and Genomics (ACMG) recommend that clinicians consider NGS when testing for genetic causes of hearing loss [56]. Prior to considering genetic testing, clinicians should

http://dx.doi.org/10.5772/61218

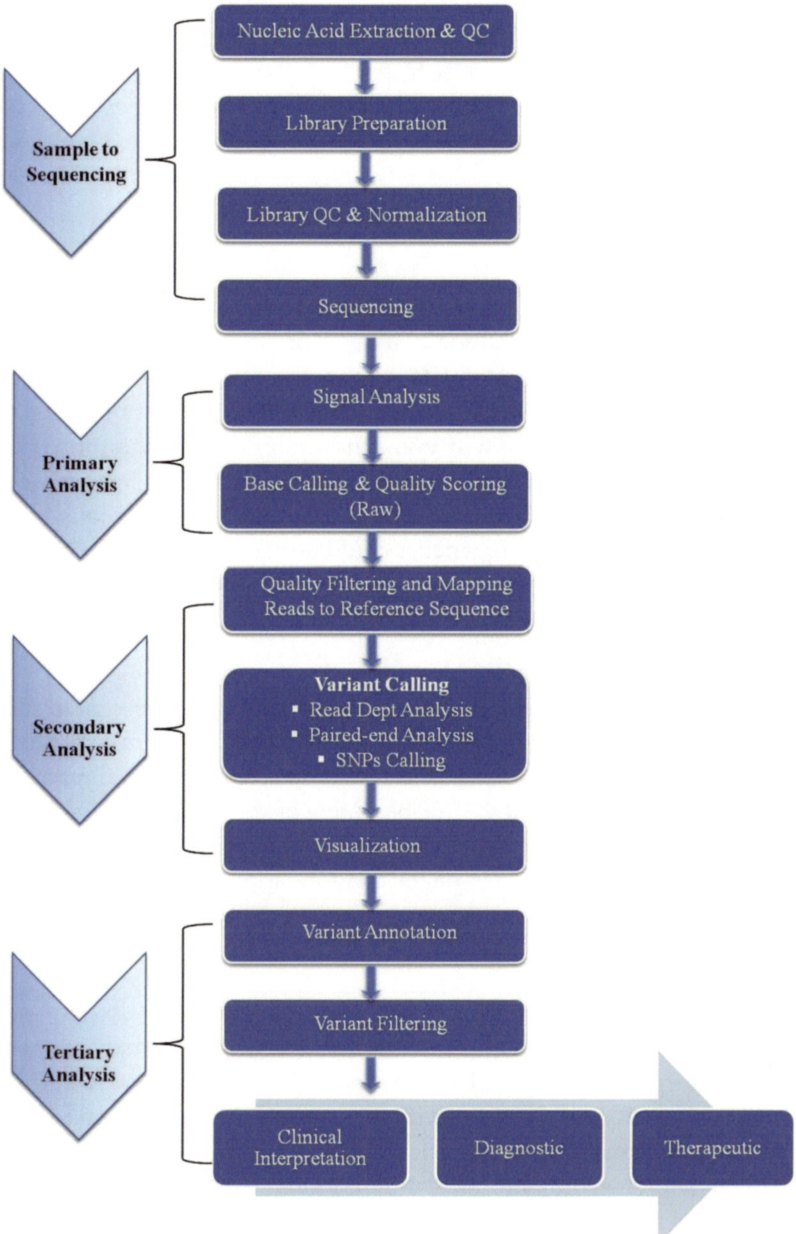

Figure 1. Next-generation sequencing: An approach from sample to analysis.

undertake a comprehensive evaluation of the patients' medical histories, including birth, that will help distinguish acquired versus inherited causes of hearing loss. They should also perform audiological evaluations to determine the type and degree of hearing loss, as recommended by ACMG. ACMG also recommends genetic testing and counseling that could include single-gene tests, panels, genome/exome sequencing, chromosome analysis, and array-based copy number analysis if clinical findings suggest syndromic genetic hearing loss. Single-gene testing may be needed if medical and family history suggests non-syndromic hearing loss that is not associated with environmental causes. If none is suggested, the next step could be *GJB2* or *GJB6* testing. If single-gene tests yield no diagnosis, clinicians may consider NGS that quickly replaces many single-gene tests for hearing loss and can assess patients whose phenotypes are not easily distinguished clinically [58].

3.2. Cytogenetics

Cytogenetic tests are a diagnostic tool for a number of clinical syndromes associated with hearing loss. They proved the causal association between specific chromosomal abnormalities and clinical features observed in patients. Although cytogenetics is not the first technique to be considered when evaluating a child with non-syndromic deafness, this form of testing could be valuable in cases of deafness of unknown etiology, particularly if there were accompanying congenital anomalies, or a family history of multiple spontaneous abortions. When all other causes of deafness are eliminated, cytogenetics could be used to determine if the hearing loss may be due to a chromosome rearrangement, such as a balanced translocation. The advantage would be that, if such a chromosome rearrangement were found, it would immediately suggest the location of the deafness gene [59].

Cytogenetic or molecular cytogenetic tests such as karyotyping, fluorescent in situ hybridization (FISH), or chromosomal microarray analysis (CMA) may provide diagnostic information when syndromes characterized by chromosomal aneuploidies, structural rearrangements, or deletions or duplications are suspected. Genetic testing of specific individual genes (PAX3 for Waardenburg syndromes types I and III), or small panels of genes related to a specific clinical finding (FGFR-related craniosynostosis panel) may be appropriate, depending on the suspected diagnosis [60].

3.2.1. Prenatal diagnosis

Prenatal diagnosis of chromosomal aberrations requires cytogenetic analysis of amniotic fetal cells. Amniocentesis is an invasive, well-established, safe, and reliable test during pregnancy that removes a small amount of fluid from the sac around the baby to look for birth defects and chromosomal problems. Amniocentesis is done from 12 to 15 weeks of gestation for chromosomal analysis. When the amniotic sample is received in the laboratory, it is centrifuged at 750 rpm for 10 minutes. The amniotic fluid is then carefully decanted from the cell pellet into a sterile test tube, and then the cell pellet is re-suspended in amniotic fluid. Then, suitable medium supplemented with fetal bovine serum, L-glutamine, and antibiotics are added and the cultures are incubated at 37ºC in 5% CO_2 incubator. The cells are harvested at 8-10 days after culture, subjected to routine hypotonic and fixative treatments as for whole blood culture, and then the chromosomes are analyzed [61].

Genetic screening for a specific mitochondrial mutation during pregnancy could offer a strategy of minimizing hearing loss in babies from exposure to avoidable risk factors such as neonatal use of aminoglycoside antibiotics [3]. Genetic counseling should ideally be offered to all pregnant women who have a family history of any condition that might be tested by either amniocentesis or chorionic villus sampling (CVS). It is important to offer genetic counseling before and after prenatal diagnostic testing. The important aspects should be considered such as presentation of the background risk of congenital disease and anomaly, and individual increased risks (such as increased maternal age), options and limitations for prenatal genetic diagnosis, possible diseases that can be detected, risks associated with the relevant tests, and conflictual areas in relation to prenatal diagnosis and alternatives. [62]. Different techniques used in genetic analysis and their applications are summarized in Table 7.

Techniques	Applications	Year, Discovered/ Reported by	References
Sanger Sequencing	Sequencing of targeted genes to analyze variations	1975, Frederick Sanger	[63]
FISH (fluorescence in situ hybridization)	Detect and localize the presence or absence of specific DNA sequences on chromosomes	1980, Bauman et al.	[64]
RFLP (Restriction Fragment Length Polymorphism)	Variations in homologous DNA sequences	1984, Sir Alec Jeffreys	[65]
Microarray	Copy number variation of numbers of genes involved in disease	1995, Schena et al.	[66]
qRT-PCR	Copy number variations of targeted genes	1996, Heid et al.	[67]
SMRT (Single molecule real time sequencing)	Detects variations of entire genome and/or coding regions, genome resequencing, transcriptome profiling, DNA-protein interactions, maximum read length >40,000 bases	2003, Levene et al.	[68]
Clinical exome sequencing	Analyzes the exons or coding regions of thousands of genes simultaneously	2009, Sarah B Ng et al.	[69]

Table 7. Different techniques used in genetic analysis and applications.

Molecular genetic testing can be helpful because an etiology cannot be otherwise established in the majority of individuals with genetic hearing loss. Molecular analysis is essentially non-invasive and may reduce the need for more extensive and expensive testing; it sometimes requires sedation or general anesthesia of infants and children. Molecular analysis can be beneficial for the diagnosis of syndromic hearing loss before additional features emerge (e.g., in Pendred syndrome or Jervell and Lange-Nielsen syndrome), and can distinguish individuals with mitochondrial mutations who are at risk for iatrogenic hearing loss when treated with aminoglycosides [4]. There are other benefits of molecular analysis, which include associated knowledge of the pattern of inheritance and more accurate genetic counseling. Recently developed high-throughput techniques reduce the burden of the costs of sequencing.

For example, sequencing costs have massively reduced from $5,292.39/Mb in 2001 to $0.06/Mb by April 2013 [70]. It is estimated that the sequencing costs will further reduce with precipitous dropping per-base cost with advancing techniques.

3.3. Limitations and challenges

Despite the significant advantages of genetic testing, there are also several limitations and challenges. These limitations and challenges are briefly discussed below:

- The spectrum of DNA variation in a human genome comprises small base changes (substitutions), insertions and deletions of DNA, large genomic deletions of exons or whole genes, and rearrangements such as inversions and translocations. Traditional Sanger sequencing is restricted to the discovery of substitutions and small insertions and deletions [71].
- Although NGS promises a personalized approach to complex diseases, it has limitations. NGS cannot detect large deletions or duplications of DNA or nucleotide repeats that can cause disease. These limitations of NGS technologies may necessitate use of alternative or complementary genetic testing strategies in some cases.
- Not all regions of the genome are efficiently captured and analyzed by current exon-capture or WGS approaches, and large deletions and duplications, in addition to copy-number and structural variations, may not be efficiently detected [72].
- It is possible to determine with recent technology if an asymptomatic newborn has a mutation in the genes known to be implicated to hearing loss, although there is no certainty that all of these genes will be responsible for the incidence of hearing loss in the future.
- Current methods of DNA analysis require 2-5 mls of blood, which would be unacceptable for a newborn screen. However, It is anticipated that sufficient DNA could be extracted from a drop of blood collected for newborn bloodspot metabolic screen, with improved sequence techniques (the Guthrie test) [3].
- Genetic testing for deafness is not collectively perceived to be advantageous. Deafness is not usually considered to be negative or limiting especially by the deaf community. Many deaf individuals consider themselves to be part of their own linguistic (sign language) and cultural group, where they have their own values, identity, and traditions. It is not perceived to be a medical condition or disability. As a result, advances in hearing loss research and genetic testing might be perceived as harmful. Genetic services may be considered; however, some individuals prefer to have deaf children [4, 73].
- A positive genetic test can also lead to an increased level of anxiety and individuals may feel guilty for having potentially passed a gene alteration on to their children.

4. Development and evaluation of genetic treatment for hearing loss

Despite recent developments in medicine, there is still no cure for most types of hearing loss. The development of a biological method for the repair, regeneration, and replacement of hair cells of the damaged cochlea has the potential to restore normal hearing. At present, gene therapy and stem cells are two promising therapeutic applications for hearing disorders.

4.1. Gene therapy

Gene therapy involves using specific sequences of DNA to treat human disease. It is an experimental form of treatment that is still being developed, but it has a unique application for hearing loss. Two main gene therapy approaches have been considered: replacing a mutated gene that causes disorder with a healthy copy of the gene, or inactivating a mutated gene that is functioning improperly. Gene therapy technology has improved in recent years, making it a promising technique for treating hearing disorders. The gene vector, the route of gene administration, the therapeutic gene, and the target cells are four major elements of gene therapy. With the recent developments in the field, a wide variety of viral and non-viral vectors have emerged that can deliver genetic payloads to target cells in the inner ear. There are three viral vectors commonly utilized for gene therapy (targeted at the inner ear): adenoviral vectors, adeno-associated viral vectors, and lentiviral vectors. Several promising clinical trials have been reported using gene therapy.

The first study of gene therapy for hearing disorders was reported in 1994 by Fujiyoshi and colleagues. They developed the myelin basic protein (MBP) transgenic mice by microinjecting an MBP cosmid clone into the pronucleus of fertilized eggs of shiverer mice to replace the autosomal recessive mutation (deletion) gene by the transgene for MBP. The MBP transgenic mice were found to recover up to 25% of normal levels of MBP, and significantly higher myelinated axons were present in the transgenic mice compare to control mice [74, 75]. In 1996, other studies reported that foreign genes were successfully transfected into the inner ear using replication-deficient viral vectors [75-77].

The discovery of RNA interference (RNAi)-mediated gene inactivation has introduced a new mechanism for targeted therapy of the inner ear at the molecular level [78]. RNAi is an intracellular two-step process that converts precursor double-stranded RNA molecules into functional small interfering RNAs (siRNAs). Synthetic double-stranded RNAs can be introduced as siRNA mimics and used to trigger RNAi and intentionally reduce the expression of targeted genes for therapeutic applications. A few allele variants of *GJB2* cause autosomal dominant non-syndromic hearing loss as a dominant-negative consequence of expression of the mutant protein. Allele-specific gene suppression by RNAi is a potentially attractive strategy to prevent hearing loss caused by this mechanism [79]. Since inheritance is autosomal dominant, silencing the mutated allele is predicted to preserve hearing. A recent proof-of-principle study validated this prediction—an siRNA was shown to potently suppress expression of the *R75W* allele of human *GJB2* in a murine model [79, 80].

Bacterial artificial chromosome (BAC) mediated transgenesis has proven to be a highly reliable way to obtain accurate transgene expression for in vivo studies of gene expression and function. BAC transgenes direct gene expression at physiological levels with the same developmental timing and expression patterns as endogenous genes in transgenic animal models. Recently, transgene expression through the germline was demonstrated to maintain normal inner ear morphology and stable hearing function in a mouse model of human non-syndromic deafness DFNB3 caused by a missense mutation in the *Myo15a* gene on mouse chromosome 11. In addition, excess *Myo15a* expression has no physiologically significant protective or deleterious effects on hearing of normal mice, suggesting that the dosage of *Myo15a* may not be problematic for gene therapy [80, 81].

Neurotrophic factors are essential in the development of the inner ear and are able to protect inner ear hair cells and spiral ganglion neurons from the damage caused by various pathogenic factors and promote the recovery from cochlear injury. Up to now, more than 20 neurotrophic factors have been revealed with protective effects on inner ear cells [75]. Neurotrophin gene therapy is promising both in the protection against exogenous damage and the regeneration after endogenous and exogenous damage. It has been reported that neurotrophic factors, such as BDNF (brain-derived neurotrophic factor), NT-3 (neurotrophins 3), TGF (transforming growth factor), GDNF (glial cell line-derived neurotrophic factor), FGF (fibroblast growth factor), CNTF (ciliary neurotrophic factor), and HGF (hepatocyte growth factor) have protective effects of different extents on inner ear hair cells and neurons [82-86].

The discovery of new therapies for the treatment of hereditary hearing loss will depend on a better understanding of gene function in the survival and differentiation of existing neurons, and encourages the growth and differentiation of new neurons and synapses, bonding nerves to cochlear hair cells to form synaptic connections as well as in maintaining the unique inner ear ion balance.

Atoh1 (Math1) gene acts as a "switch" to turn on hair cell growth and it is discovered that *Atoh1* is artificially switched on in the cells that support hair cells (called "supporting cells"); it instructs them to divide and form new hair cells. *Atoh1 (Math1)* plays an important role in the differentiation of hair cells of the developing inner ear and restore auditory function [87-89]. Using the tools of gene therapy may activate *Atoh1* to induce undamaged cells within the cochlea to develop into hair cells in an adult human ear and rebuild a damaged ear by replicating the steps that took place during embryonic development. There is still a lot of work to be done for human adult ear. *CGF-166* gene therapy has been shown to activate the *Atoh1* biological pathway and the gene was able to safely restore hearing in animal models. Recently, the clinical trial started to test if *CGF166* will have the same beneficial effect in humans [90]. Researchers believe that this therapy would not help people with types of inherited deafness where the structures in the ear needed to support new hair cell growth are missing or those who have damaged auditory nerves.

There is no ideal gene delivery system for gene therapy so far. Three kinds of vectors (bacterial vector, multiplex gene vector, labeled gene vector) may have great prospects. Long-term human gene therapy will not be feasible until there is substantial improvement in transduction efficiencies into human tissues. The combination of more efficient gene transfers, targeted vector systems, and effective and relatively nontoxic selection systems to maintain gene expression may make the long-term correction of hearing disorders feasible and safe. Some practices of inner ear gene therapy may need to be carried out at the embryonic stage for the treatment of hereditary hearing loss in the future.

4.2. Stem cells therapy

The recent developments in stem cell technologies are opening novel therapeutic possibilities for the treatment of hearing disorders. Stem cell therapy is a relatively new technique used to treat many forms of human disease in which exogenous stem cells are used to replace dead or damaged endogenous cell types. In recent years, researchers have undertaken a number of successful animal studies in the area of developing stem cell therapies for hearing loss and able to turn stem cells into many of the cell types in the inner ear whose damage and death leads to hearing loss, such as hair cells and auditory nerve cells.

Stem cells are a group of cells in our bodies with the capacity to self-renew and differentiate to various types of cells, thus to construct tissues and organs. When a stem cell divides, each new cell has the potential either to remain undifferentiated (self-renewal) or become a specialized (differentiation) type of cell with a specific function. Stem cells can be classified into different types, based on their source of origin, the time of derivation, and the potential to produce different lineages. The primordial master stem cell is the zygote. The zygote and early blastomeres are totipotent and can generate any and all human cells type in the body, such as the brain, liver, blood, or heart cells. It can even give rise to a whole functional organism including extraembryonic tissues. Pluripotent stem cells have a slightly more limited potential. They have the ability to produce cell types from all three embryonic germ layers (endoderm, mesoderm, and ectoderm), including all the somatic lineages as well as germ cells; but infrequently, if ever, can produce extraembroynic lineages such as those from the placenta. It cannot form an entire functional organism. Lastly, multipotent stem cells such as hematopoietic stem cells have a more limited ability, producing cell types usually restricted to a single organ or germ layer. Multipotent stem cells have the ability to differentiate into a closely related family of cells. Pluripotent stem cells have the widest range of potential applications. They can generally be classified as embryonic or adult, depending on their developmental stage of derivation.

Embryonic and adult stem cells differ primarily in the number of different cells each can produce. Embryonic stem cells are derived from a four- or five-day-old embryo that is in the blastocyst phase of development. It can develop into any cell type of the body. In contrast, adult stem cells reside in many organs of the adult human body and can generate a range of cell types from the originating organ or even regenerate the entire original organ. Adult stem cells can be found in a great number of organs and tissues including the brain, bone marrow, peripheral blood, blood vessels, skeletal muscle, skin, teeth, heart, gut, liver, ovarian epithelium, and testis [91]. A relatively recent breakthrough in stem cell research is the discovery that specialized adult (somatic) cells can be 'reprogrammed' into cells that behave like embryonic stem cells, termed induced pluripotent stem cells (iPSCs) [92]. Like human embryonic stem cells, the iPS (induced pluripotent stem cells) cells are immortal, pluripotent, and express genes characteristic of all three embryonic germ cell layers (endoderm, ectoderm, and mesoderm) when induced to differentiate.

A number of criteria must be satisfied to achieve functional restoration, including generation of an adequate number of cells to invert the defects, differentiation of the cells to the correct phenotype, formation of appropriate three-dimensional tissue structures, and production of cells/tissues that are mechanically and structurally complaint with the native tissue without immunological rejection [80, 93]. The generation of neural stem cells and control of neural differentiation from human embryonic stem cells have opened new doors for therapy of hearing disorders. Several studies have demonstrated successful delivery of embryonic and adult stem cells to normal and damaged tissues in vivo, and in some cases a therapeutic effect has been observed.

One of the first reports of stem cell delivery to the inner ear was a study by Ito and colleagues (2001) that demonstrated survival and migration of adult rat hippocampus-derived neural stem cells (NSCs) implanted into the rat cochlea. Within 2-4 weeks of grafting to the cochlea, some NSCs survived in the cochlear cavity. Some of them had adopted the morphologies and positions of hair cells [94]. Following this study was a report about the potential of NSC transplantation to the damaged mouse cochlea. The majority of transplanted cells integrated in the vestibular sensory epithelia and expressed specific markers (myosin VIIa) for hair cells in vivo. The result of this study suggests that transplanted NSCs have the potential to differentiate and restore inner ear hair cells. However, a small number of hair cell marker-positive grafted cells and no evidence of synaptic connections between transplants and host spiral ganglion neurons hampered well-established methods for functional recovery [95]. The principal differences between human and mouse NSCs seem to be the length of the cell cycle (up to 4 days in humans) and the predilection of human cells to senesce (after ~100 cell divisions) [96]. NSCs can achieve therapeutic efficacy in human clinical applications, although many limitations remain to be overcome.

Several studies reported on the transplantation of embryonic stem (ES) cells into the inner ear. ES cells have the ability to differentiate into neuronal cell types when transplanted into the spiral ganglion of cochlea. ES cells that have been transplanted into the spiral ganglion of the cochlea were found to express neural markers [97, 98] and develop cellular processes similar to axons that extend towards the organ of Corti [99-102]. Some of these stem cell-derived neurons were shown to establish synaptic contacts with sensory hair cells, the peripheral target for spiral ganglion neurons (SGNs) in vitro (Matsumoto et al., 2008) and to survive in animals with selective loss of SGNs [99, 103].

For a cell therapy approach aiming at restoring impaired function, implanted cells need to be able to convey auditory information from the periphery to more centrally located nuclei. Recent studies have shown that dorsal root ganglion cells or ES cells are transplanted to the transected auditory nerve migrated along the nerve fibers in the internal auditory meatus and, in some cases, even reach proximate to the ventral cochlear nucleus in the brainstem [104, 105]. Interestingly, Ito et al. (2001) reported that embryonic brain tissue transplanted to the acutely transected ventral cochlear tract resulted in not only regeneration but additionally functional recovery [105, 106]. However, there are many chemical factors that produce a barrier between the peripheral and central nervous system and could impede the ability of central processes of replacement neurons to make a connection in the cochlear nucleus.

A number of studies have shown that adult bone marrow-derived stem cells (MSCs) can also have therapeutic potential in the damaged inner ear. MSCs have shown plasticity with a capacity to differentiate into a variety of specialized cells. MSCs have been delivered both systemically and by direct injection through the scala tympani into the mouse and gerbil cochlea respectively [107, 108]. Matsuoka and colleagues investigated the potential of MSCs to adopt properties of SGNs in vivo [108]. Identification of stem cells in the human fetal cochlea [109] contributes to the study stem cell biology of the auditory organ in humans, while advances in identification of stem cells have been made in rodents [110].

Umbilical cord blood (UCB) is the most recently identified useful source of hematopoietic stem cells (HSCs) for treatment of a wide variety of disorders. UCB has potential applications in hearing disorders. A study provided the first evidence of positive engraftment of intravenously transplanted human umbilical cord blood CD133+ HSCs into the inner ear of NOD-SCID mice rendered deaf with kanamycin and noise in vivo [111]. In another study, the researchers have demonstrated that hematopoietic stem cell transplantation (HSCT) may provide improvement in mucopolysaccharidosis-associated sensorineural hearing loss [112]. Recently, an FDA-approved clinical trial involving stem cells derived from UCB has been initiated for treatment of children with sensorineural hearing loss [113].

Mammalian cochlear hair cells do not regenerate spontaneously, although vestibular hair cells in adult mammals regenerate at levels so low as to rule out any significant functional recovery [114, 115]. The discovery of stem cells has opened the possibility of devising strategies to recruit these cells to repair damaged or lost cochlear hair cells. Stem cells are important tools for hearing disorder research and offer great potential for use in the clinic. Certain types of stem cells, such as neural stem cells, are more capable than others of replacing lost or damaged hair cells, although they have limitations. There is a great challenge in identifying more effective ways of directing stem cells to develop into inner ear hair cells. The field of auditory stem cell research is still in its infancy, although important advances are already taking place. Stem cell therapy for hearing loss is some years away from being clinically feasible.

5. Management and prevention of hereditary hearing loss

Gene therapy and stem cell treatment have still a long way to go before these treatments will be available to use in humans. Therefore, existing measures must focus on the prevention of hearing loss to decrease the frequency of genetic hearing loss. There is a need of improved implementation of genetic counseling and awareness in populations that are at high risk of hereditary hearing loss.

Early detection and intervention of hearing loss is the most important factor in minimizing the impact of hearing loss on a child's development and educational achievements. At least, all children with a risk for hereditary hearing loss need to be given screening audiometry. The hearing loss can be progressive in nature for a person with autosomal recessive non-syndromic hearing loss caused by mutations in *SLC26A4*. In such case, audiometric testing may be warranted every year. Additionally, thyroid function should be followed if the diagnosis is consistent with Pendred syndrome [14]. Sequential audiologic examinations are essential to document the stability or progression of the hearing loss and to identify and treat superimposed hearing losses, such as middle ear effusion.

Knowledge of the genetic cause is helpful in determining the kind of damage to the auditory system that caused deafness. Identification of the underlying cause in terms of how the inner ear is damaged may assist in choosing rehabilitation strategies, such as hearing aid or cochlear implant. In children with congenital severe-to-profound autosomal recessive non-syndromic hearing loss who are positive for mutations in *GJB2* and *GJB6* at the DFNB1 locus and who elect to receive cochlear implants, performance outcome is outstanding [116]. In addition, a recent cochlear implant study stated that children with identified *GJB2* mutations, which cause an isolated insult to the cochlea without damage to the 8th nerve or the central auditory system, benefitted from cochlear implantation in the areas of speech production, speech perception, and language [4].

5.1. Genetic counseling

Genetic counseling is an important part of evaluation and management of hearing disorders. The process of genetic counseling is intended to inform patients and their families of the medical, psychological, and familial implications of genetic hearing disorders, as well as the risks, benefits, and limitations of genetic testing. In the United States, genetics professionals recommend "non-directive" counseling. It is meant to be informative and supportive rather than advise people what to do or whether or not to have children. Genetic information can help predict whether the hearing loss will remain the same or whether it will worsen over time. In addition, genetic testing can help determine if problems besides hearing loss may be present or may develop in the future. It can also help patients and families who may be at risk for conditions that can be passed down in families (inherited conditions). There are a number of people who may have quite different attitudes about deafness in their family. Some hearing parents might be concerned about having another deaf child, while others may believe that the hearing loss would not cause a problem, but they would want to know if any other associated medical problems might be involved. Likewise, deaf parents may feel comfortable about their own abilities, but would have a better opinion of not to have a deaf child, in view of the fact that other deaf parents may be more worried about the challenges of raising a hearing child [117]. In such case, the genetic counselor should be very cautious in providing information concerning the nature of the disease, the implications of being carriers (mutation carriers of genes associated with hearing loss), and the reproductive choices. Genetic counseling services for families with deafness can only be effective and appropriate if the social values of the deaf community are taken into consideration.

6. Conclusions and future perspectives

Advances in genetic testing are already directly impacting people's lives. The demand for molecular tests is by now increasing with the discovery of the varied molecular defects underlying hearing loss. Genetic testing has now reached a stage where it is becoming increasingly applicable for precise diagnosis of hearing disorders. The development of NGS technology has made DNA sequencing not only rapid and cost-effective, but also highly accurate and reproducible. In the near future, it is expected that there will be more enhancements in the speed and cost of DNA sequencing. We are already in the modern DNA sequencing era, where aims of third- and fourth-generation DNA sequencing additionally boost the speed of sequencing and reduce costs. Although sequencing the whole genome seems exhaustive, it could be more cost-effective than having to select the genes of interest [118]. Once genome sequencing becomes more cost-effective and fast, it will accelerate the pace of gene discovery for deafness and clinical application of this discovery will be realized. Over the next few years, most molecular genetic testing will be performed on automated instruments and some genetic tests for hearing disorders will be available as at-home kits on a large scale.

One of the roles of genetic testing is to identify presently known genetic causes of hearing loss in failed hearing screening of newborns and children who are identified with childhood-onset hearing loss. Furthermore, it increases our knowledge of the genetic causes of hearing loss. The potential for increased usage of aminoglycoside antibiotics also supports the case for a genetic screening program of pregnant women for the *m.1555A G* mutation, which could avoid unnecessary cases of hearing loss. Only when a reliable estimate of the future risks of hearing loss can be made at a reasonable cost will genetic screening become viable [3].

Molecular diagnostic results should always be interpreted with caution, as our knowledge of the molecular basis of hearing loss is still evolving. Keeping pace with emerging clinical genetic technologies requires specialized genetic training as well as broad genetic literacy for patients and clinicians ordering and receiving genetics test results. Genetic information that is shared by the patient and patient's family is unique. The application of genetic tests has appropriately generated substantial debate in the community with regard to the delivery and impact of the information on clinicians, patients, and society in general. The potential for misuse of genetic information is enormous and requires action to protect the privacy of genetic information and protect individuals from discrimination based on genetic information. The ethical, legal, and social issues surrounding genetic testing for hearing loss need to be addressed. In the near future, more studies of the ethical and social aspects of genetic testing for hearing disorders should be done. It is hoped that the potential for misuse of genetic information in the future will be limited.

Some of the novel rehabilitation options under development to slow down the progression of hearing loss are gene and even mutation specific [80], suggesting that comprehensive genetic testing will be an integral part of the care of deaf and hard-of-hearing patients in the future [9]. Over time, the genetic diagnostic tests will become available faster, followed by targeted gene therapy or various permutations of progenitor cell transplantation, and eventually, the preventive interventions for a wider range of hearing impaired patients.

Author details

Sidheshwar Pandey[1*] and Mukeshwar Pandey[2]

*Address all correspondence to: sidheshwarp@yahoo.co.in

1 DRETCHI, Trinidad and Tobago Association for the Hearing Impaired, Port of Spain, Trinidad and Tobago, West Indies

2 Premas Lifescience, a division of Premas Biotech Pvt Ltd, New Delhi, India

References

[1] Friedman TB, Griffith AJ. Human nonsyndromic sensorineural deafness. Annu Rev Genomics Hum Genet. 2003;4:341-402.

[2] Hilgert N, Smith RJ, Van Camp G. Forty six genes causing non-syndromic hearing impairment: Which ones should be analysed in DNA diagnostics? Mutat Res. 2009;681:189-196.

[3] Linden Phillips L, Bitner-Glindzicz M, Lench N, et al. The future role of genetic screening to detect newborns at risk of childhood-onset hearing loss. Inter J Audiolo 2013;52:124-133.

[4] Schrijver, I. Hereditary non-syndromic sensorineural hearing loss: Transforming silence to sound. The Journal of Molecular Diagnostics: JMD. 2004;6:275-284.

[5] Guilford P, Ben Arab S, Blanchard S, Levilliers J, Weissenbach J, Belkahia A and Petit C. A non-syndrome form of neurosensory, recessive deafness maps to the pericentromeric region of chromosome 13q. Nat Genet. 1994;6:24-8.

[6] Mahdieh N, Rabbani B, Inoue, I. Genetics of Hearing Loss, In: Dr. SadafNaz. Hearing Loss. (Ed.). InTech; 2012. ISBN: 978-953-51-0366-0, DOI: 10.5772/31984.

[7] Smith RJ, Bale JF Jr, White KR. Sensorineural hearing loss in children. Lancet. 2005;365:879-890.

[8] Van Camp G, Willems PJ, Smith RJ. Nonsyndromic hearing impairment: Unparalleled heterogeneity. Am J Hum Genet. 1997;60:758-764.

[9] Shearer AE, Deluca AP, Hildebrand MS, Taylor KR, Gurrola J, Scherer S, et al. Comprehensive genetic testing for hereditary hearing loss using massively parallel sequencing. In: Proceedings of the National Academy of Sciences of the United States of America. 2010;107:21104-21109.

[10] Van Camp G, Smith RJH. Hereditary Hearing Loss Homepage. 2014. Available from: http://www.hereditaryhearingloss.org [Accessed: 2015-01-27].

[11] Kelsell DP, Dunlop J, Stevens HP, Lench NJ, Liang JN, Parry G, Mueller RF, Leigh IM. Connexin 26 mutations in hereditary non-syndromic sensorineural deafness. Nature. 1997;387:80-3.

[12] Nie L. *KCNQ4* mutations associated with non-syndromic progressive sensorineural hearing loss. Curr Opin Otolaryngol Head Neck Surg. 2008;16:441-4.

[13] Hildebrand MS, Tack D, McMordie S, DeLuca A, Ae Hur I, Nishimura C, Huygen P, Casavant TL, Smith RJH. Audioprofile-directed screening identifies novel mutations in KCNQ4 causing hearing loss at the DFNA2 locus. Genet Med. 2008;10:797-804.

[14] Smith RJH, Shearer AE, Hildebrand MS, and Camp VG. Deafness and Hereditary Hearing Loss Overview. In: Pagon RA, Adam MP, Ardinger HH, et al., editors GeneReviews®. Seattle (WA): University of Washington, Seattle; 1993-2015. Available from: http://www.ncbi.nlm.nih.gov/books/NBK1434/.

[15] Smith RJ, Hone S. Genetic screening for deafness. Pediatr Clin North Am. 2003;50:315-29.

[16] Chan DK, Chang KW. GJB2-associated hearing loss: Systematic review of worldwide prevalence, genotype, and auditory phenotype. Laryngoscope. 2014;124:E34-53.

[17] Grifa A, Wagner CA, D'Ambrosio L, Melchionda S, Bernardi F, Lopez-Bigas N, Rabionet R, Arbones M, Monica MD, Estivill X, Zelante L, Lang F, Gasparini P. Mutations in GJB6 cause nonsyndromic autosomal dominant deafness at DFNA3 locus. Nat Genet. 1999;23:16-18.

[18] Del Castillo I, Villamar M, Moreno-Pelayo MA, del Castillo FJ, Alvarez A, Telleria D, Menendez I, Moreno F. A deletion involving the connexin 30 gene in nonsyndromic hearing impairment. N Engl J Med. 2002;346:243-249.

[19] Bayazit YA, Yilmaz M. An overview of hereditary hearing loss. *ORL* J Otorhinolaryngol Relat Spec. 2006;68:57-63.

[20] Rost S, Bach E, Neuner, Nanda I, Dysek S, Bittner RE, et al. Novel form of X-linked nonsyndromic hearing loss with cochlear malformation caused by a mutation in the type IV collagen gene COL4A6. European J Human Genet. 2014;22:208-215.

[21] Jacobs H T, Hutchin T P, Kappi T, Gillies G, Minkkinen K, Walker J, et al. Mitochondrial DNA mutations in patients with postlingual, nonsyndromic hearing impairment. Eur. J. Hum. Genet. 2005;13:26-33.

[22] Filosto M, Mancuso M. Mitochondrial diseases: A nosological update. Acta Neurologica Scandinavica. 2007;115:211-221.

[23] Scarpelli M, Zappini F, Filosto M, Russignan A, Tonin P, Tomelleri G. Mitochondrial sensorineural hearing loss: A retrospective study and a description of cochlear im-

plantation in a melas patient, Genetics Research International, vol. 2012, Article ID 287432, 5 pages, 2012. DOI: 10.1155/2012/287432.

[24] Tang X, Yang L, Zhu Y, Liao Z, Wang J, Qian Y, Tao Z, Hu L, Wu G, Lan J, Wang X, Ji J, Wu J, Ji Y, Feng J, Chen J, Li Z, Zhang X, Lu J, Guan M-X. Very low penetrance of hearing loss in seven Han Chinese pedigrees carrying the deafness-associated 12S rRNA A1555G mutation. Gene. 2007;393:11-19.

[25] Prezant TR, Agapian JV, Bohlman MC et al. Mitochondrial ribosomal RNA mutation associated with both antibiotic-induced and non-syndromic deafness. Nat Genet. 1993;4:289-294.

[26] Estivill X, Govea N, Barcelo A, et al. Familial progressive sensorineural deafness is mainly due to the mtDNA A1555G mutation and is enhanced by treatment with aminoglycosides. American J Human Genet. 1998;62:27-35.

[27] Pandya A. Non-syndromic hearing loss and deafness. In: Pagon RA, Adam MP, Ardinger HH, et al., editors. Mitochondrial. Seattle (WA): University of Washington, Seattle. GeneReviews®; 2014; 1993-2015.

[28] Chamber HF, Sande MA. The aminoglycosides. In: The Pharmocological Basis of Therapeutic. Hardman JG, Limbird LE, Molinoff PB, Ruddon RW, Gilman A, editors. 9th edition. New York. McGraw-Hill; 1996. pp.1103-1221.

[29] Kokotas H, Petersen MB and Willems PJ. Mitochondrial deafness. Clin Genet. 2007;71: 379-391.

[30] Scarpelli M, Zappini F, Filosto M, Russignan A, Tonin P, Tomelleri G. Mitochondrial sensorineural hearing loss: A retrospective study and a description of cochlear implantation in a melas patient. Genet Res. Inter. 2012; p5 DOI: 10.1155/2012/287432.

[31] Sinnathuray AR, Raut V, Awa A, Magee A, Toner JG. A review of cochlear implantation in mitochondrial sensorineural hearing loss. Otology and Neurotology. 2003;24:418-426.

[32] Toriello HV, Reardon W, Gorlin RJ. Hereditary hearing loss and its syndromes 2nd ed. New York: Oxford University Press; 2004.

[33] Huang BY, Zdanski C, Castillo M. Pediatric Sensorineural Hearing Loss, Part 2: Syndromic and Acquired Causes. AJNR Am J Neuroradiol. 2012;33:399-406.

[34] Lunardi S, Forli F, Michelucci A, Liumbruno A, Baldinotti F, Fogli A, Bertini V, Valetto A, Toschi B, Simi P, Boldrini A, Berrettini S, Ghirri P. Genetic Hearing Loss Associated with Craniofacial Abnormalities, Hearing Loss. In: Dr. Sadaf Naz (Ed.), InTech; 2012. ISBN: 978-953-51-0366-0.

[35] Putcha GV, Bejjani BA, Bleoo S, Booker JK, Carey JC, Carson N, et al. A multicenter study of the frequency and distribution of GJB2 and GJB6 mutations in a large North American cohort. Genet. Med. 2007;9:413-426.

[36] De Keulenaer et al. Molecular diagnostics for congenital hearing loss including 15 deafness genes using a next generation sequencing platform. BMC Med. Genomics. 2012;5:17.

[37] Brown KK, Rehm HL. Molecular diagnosis of hearing loss. Curr Protoc Hum Genet. 2012;72:9.16.1-9.16.16.

[38] Sirmaci A, Edwards YJ, Akay H, Tekin M. Challenges in whole exome sequencing: An example from hereditary deafness. PLoS ONE 2012;7:e32000.

[39] Alford RL, Arnos KS, Fox M, Lin JW, Palmer CG, Pandya A, Rehm HL, Robin NH, Scott DA, Yoshinaga-Itano C. American College of Medical Genetics and Genomics guideline for the clinical evaluation and etiologic diagnosis of hearing loss. Genetics in Medicine. 2014;16:347-355. DOI: 10.1038/gim.2014.2

[40] Summerer D. Enabling technologies of genomic-scale sequence enrichment for targeted high-throughput sequencing. Genomics. 2009;94:363-368.

[41] Turner EH. Ng SB. Nickerson DA, et al. Methods for genomic partitioning. Annu Rev Genomics Hum Genet. 2009;10:263-284.

[42] Mamanova L. Coffey AJ. Scott CE, et al. Target-enrichment strategies for next-generation sequencing. Nat Methods. 2010;7:111-118.

[43] Okou DT. Steinberg KM. Middle C, et al. Microarray-based genomic selection for high-throughput resequencing. Nat Methods. 2007;4:907-909.

[44] Gnirke A. Melnikov A. Maguire J, et al. Solution hybrid selection with ultra-long oligonucleotides for massively parallel targeted sequencing. Nat Biotechnol. 2009;27:182-189.

[45] Shearer AE. Hildebrand MS. Sloan CM, et al. Deafness in the genomics era. Hear Res. 2011;282:1-9.

[46] Lin X. Tang W. Ahmad S, et al. Applications of targeted gene capture and next-generation sequencing technologies in studies of human deafness and other genetic disabilities. Hear Res. 2012;288:67-76.

[47] Yan D, Tekin M, Blanton SH, Liu XZ. Next-generation sequencing in genetic hearing loss. Genetic Testing and Molecular Biomarkers. 2013;17:581-587. DOI :10.1089/gtmb. 2012.0464.

[48] Rehman AU, Morell RJ, Belyantseva IA, et al. Targeted capture and next-generation sequencing identifies C9orf75, encoding taperin, as the mutated gene in nonsyndromic deafness DFNB79. Am J Hum Genet. 2010;86:378-388.

[49] Walsh T, Shahin H, Elkan-Miller T, et al. Whole exome sequencing and homozygosity mapping identify mutation in the cell polarity protein GPSM2 as the cause of nonsyndromic hearing loss DFNB82. Am J Hum Genet. 2010; 87:90-94.

[50] Yariz KO, Duman D, Seco CZ, et al. Mutations in OTOGL, encoding the inner ear protein otogelin-like, cause moderate sensorineural hearing loss. Am J Hum Genet. 2012;91:872-882.

[51] Zheng J, Miller KK, Yang T, et al. Carcinoembryonic antigen-related cell adhesion molecule 16 interacts with alpha-tectorin and is mutated in autosomal dominant hearing loss (DFNA4) Proc Natl Acad Sci. 2011;108:4218-4223.

[52] Yan D, Zhu Y, Walsh T, et al. Mutation of the ATP-gated P2X2 receptor leads to progressive hearing loss and increased susceptibility to noise. Proc Natl Acad Sci. 2013;110:2228-2233.

[53] Schraders M, Haas SA, Weegerink NJD, et al. Next-generation sequencing identifies mutations of SMPX, which encodes the small muscle protein, X-linked, as a cause of progressive hearing impairment. Am J Hum Genet. 2011;88:628-634.

[54] Pierce SB, Walsh T, Chisholm KM, et al. Mutations in the DBP-deficiency protein HSD17B4 cause ovarian dysgenesis, hearing loss, and ataxia of Perrault syndrome. Am J Hum Genet. 2010;87:282-288.

[55] Pierce SB, Chisholm KM, Lynch ED, et al. Mutations in mitochondrial histidyl tRNA synthetase HARS2 cause ovarian dysgenesis and sensorineural hearing loss of Perrault syndrome. Proc Natl Acad Sci. 2011;108:6543-6548.

[56] Sirmaci A, Walsh T, Akay H, et al. MASP1 mutations in patients with facial, umbilical, coccygeal, and auditory findings of Carnevale, Malpuech, OSA, and Michels syndromes. Am J Hum Genet. 2010;87:679-686.

[57] Klein CJ, Botuyan MV, Wu Y, et al. Mutations in DNMT1 cause hereditary sensory neuropathy with dementia and hearing loss. Nat Genet. 2011;43:595-600.

[58] Levenson D. New testing guidelines for hearing loss support next-generation sequencing. Am. J. Med. Genet. 2014;164:7-8. DOI: 10.1002/ajmg.a.36643

[59] Anne B, Skvorak G, Cynthia C, Morton. Cytogenetics and Cochlear Expressed Sequence Tags (ESTs) for Identification of Genes Involved in Hearing and Deafness. In: Keats, Bronya J.B., Fay, Richard R. editors. Genetics of Auditory Disorders. Springer Handbook of Auditory Research. 2002; pp. 92-120. ISBN: 978-0-387-21853-3

[60] Helga VT, Shelley S. Hereditary Hearing Loss and Its Syndromes. Chapter 5: Syndrome diagnosis and investigation in the hearing impaired patient. Oxford University Press. 2013; p89.

[61] Ponnuraj KT. Cytogenetic Techniques in Diagnosing Genetic Disorders, Advances in the Study of Genetic Disorders. In: Dr. Kenji Ikehara Editor. InTech. 2011; ISBN: 978-953-307-305-7, DOI: 10.5772/17481.

[62] Wieacker P, Steinhard J. The Prenatal Diagnosis of Genetic Diseases. Deutsches Arzteblatt Inter. 2010;107:857-862. DOI: 10.3238/arztebl.2010.0857.

[63] Sanger F, Alan RC. A rapid method for determining sequences in DNA by primed synthesis with DNA polymerase. J Mol. Biol. 1975;94: 441-448

[64] Bauman JG, Wiegant J, Borst P. van Duijn P. A new method for fluorescence microscopical localization of specific DNA sequences by in situ hybridization of fluorochromelabelled RNA. Exp. Cell Res. 1980;128:485-490.

[65] Jeffreys A, Wilson V, Thein S. Hypervariable 'minisatellite' regions in human DNA. Nature. 1985;314:67-73. DOI: 10.1038/314067a0.

[66] Schena, M et al. Quantitative monitoring of gene expression patterns with a complementary DNA microarray. Sci. 1995;270: 467-470.

[67] Heid CA et al. Real time quantitative PCR. Genome Res.1996;6:986-994.

[68] Levene MJ, Korlach J, Turner SW, Foquet M, Craighead G. W.W. Webb, Zero-Mode Waveguides for Single-Molecule Analysis at high concentrations. Sci. 2003;299:682-686.

[69] Ng SB, Turner EH, Robertson PD, Flygare SD, Bigham AW, Lee C, Shaffer T, Wong M, Bhattacharjee A, Eichler EE, Bamshad M, Nickerson DA, Shendure J; Turner; Robertson; Flygare; Bigham; Lee; Shaffer; Wong; et al. "Targeted capture and massively parallel sequencing of 12 human exomes". Nature. 2009;461:272-276.

[70] Spurdle AB, Lakhani SR, Da Silva LM, Balleine RL, kConFab Investigators, et al. Bayes analysis provides evidence of pathogenicity for the BRCA1 c.135-1G>T (IVS3-1) and BRCA2 c. 7977-1G>C (IVS17-1) variants displaying in vitro splicing results of equivocal clinical significance. Hum Mutat. 2010;31:1141-1145.

[71] Behjati S, Tarpey PS. What is next generation sequencing? Archives of Disease in Childhood. Education and Practice Edition. 2013;98:236-238. DOI: 10.1136/archdischild-2013-304340.

[72] Rehm HL, Bale SJ, Bayrak-Toydemir P, et al. Working Group of the American College of Medical Genetics and Genomics Laboratory Quality Assurance Committee. ACMG clinical laboratory standards for next-generation sequencing. Genet Med. 2013;15:733-747.

[73] Middleton A, Hewison J, Mueller RF. Attitudes of deaf adults toward genetic testing for hereditary deafness. Am J Hum Genet. 1998;63:1175-1180.

[74] Fujiyoshi T, Hood L, Yoo TJ. Restoration of brain stem auditory-evoked potentials by gene transfer in shiverer mice. Ann. Otol. Rhinol. Laryngol. 1994;103:449-456.

[75] Sun H, Huang A, Cao S. Current Status and Prospects of Gene Therapy for the Inner Ear. Human Gene Therapy. 2011;22:1311-1322. DOI: 10.1089/hum.2010.246.

[76] Lalwani AK, Walsh BJ, Reilly PG, et al. Development of in vivo gene therapy for hearing disorders: Introduction of adeno-associated virus into the cochlea of the guinea pig. Gene Ther. 1996;3:588-592.

[77] Raphael Y, Frisancho JC, Roessler BJ. Adenoviral-mediated gene transfer into guinea pig cochlear cells in vivo. Neurosci Lett. 1996;207:137-141.

[78] Fire A, Xu S, Montgomery MK, Kostas SA, Driver SE, Mello CC. Potent and specific genetic interference by double-stranded RNA in,*Caenorhabditis elegans*. Nature. 1998;391:806-811.

[79] Maeda Y, Fukushima K, Nishizaki K Smith RJ. *In vitro* and *in vivo* suppression of GJB2 expression by RNA interference. Hum Mol Genet. 2005;14:1641-1650.

[80] Hildebrand MS, Newton SS, Gubbels SP, Sheffield AM, Kochhar A, De Silva MG, Dahl HH, Rose SD, Behlke MA, Smith RJ. Advances in Molecular and Cellular Therapies for Hearing Loss. Molecular Therapy. 2007;16:224-236. DOI: 10.1038/sj.mt. 6300351.

[81] Kanzaki S, Beyer L, Karolyi IJ, Dolan DF, Fang Q, Probst FJ, et al. Transgene correction maintains normal cochlear structure and function in 6-month-old Myo15a mutant mice. Hear Res. 2006;214:37-44.

[82] Staecker H, Kopke R, Malgrange B, et al. NT-3 and/or BDNF therapy prevents loss of auditory neurons following loss of hair cells. Neuroreport. 1996;7:889-894.

[83] Pickles JO, Harter C, Rebillard G. Fibroblast growth factor receptor expression in outer hair cells of rat cochlea. Neuroreport. 1998;9:4093-4095.

[84] Stover T, Yagi M, Raphael Y. Transduction of the contralateral ear after adenovirus-mediated cochlear gene transfer. Gene Ther. 2000;7:377-383.

[85] Kawamoto K, Yagi M, Stover T, et al. Hearing and hair cells are protected by adenoviral gene therapy with TGF-β_1 and GDNF. Mol. Ther. 2003;7:484-492.

[86] Nakaizumi T, Kawamoto K, Minoda R, Raphael Y. Adenovirus-mediated expression of brain-derived neurotrophic factor protects spiral ganglion neurons from ototoxic damage. Audiol. Neurootol. 2004;9:135-143.

[87] Bermingham NA, Hassan BA, Price SD, Vollrath MA, Ben-Arie N, Eatock RA, et al. Math1: An essential gene for the generation of inner ear hair cells. Sci. 1999;284: 1837-1841.

[88] Kawamoto K, Ishimoto S, Minoda R, Brough DE Raphael Y. Math1 gene transfer generates new cochlear hair cells in mature guinea pigs *in vivo*. J Neurosci. 2003;23: 4395-4400.

[89] Izumikawa M, Minoda R, Kawamoto K, Abrashkin KA, Swiderski DL, Dolan DF, et al. Auditory hair cell replacement and hearing improvement by Atoh1 gene therapy in deaf mammals. Nat Med. 2005;11:271-276.

[90] Jarvis LM. Sound Science. Emerging technology and a wide-open market are spurring more companies to pursue drugs to treat or prevent hearing loss. Chemical &

Engineering News. 2014;92. pp. 12-17. http://cen.acs.org/articles/92/i14/Sound-Science.html.

[91] Rivolta MN. Stem cells in the inner ear: Advancing towards a new therapy for hearing impairment. In: Martini A, Stephens D, Read AP. Genes, Hearing, and Deafness: From Molecular Biology to Clinical Practice. CRC Press; 2007. p. 279.

[92] Takahashi K, Tanabe K, Ohnuki M, Narita M, Ichisaka T, Tomoda K, Yamanaka S. Induction of pluripotent stem cells from adult human fibroblasts by defined factors. Cell. 2007;131: 861-872.

[93] Vats A, Tolley NS, Polak JM, Buttery LDK. Stem cells: Sources and applications. Clinical Otolaryngology & Allied Sciences. 2002;27:227-232. DOI: 10.1046/j.1365-2273.2002.00579.x.

[94] Ito J, Kojima K, Kawaguchi S. Survival of neural stem cells in the cochlea. Acta Otolaryngol. 2001;121:140-2.

[95] Tateya I, Nakagawa T, Iguchi F, Kim TS, Endo T, Yamada S, Kageyama R, Naito Y, Ito J. Fate of neural stem cells grafted into injured inner ears of mice. Neuroreport. 2003;15:1677-81.

[96] Jandial R, Singec I, Ames CP and Snyder EY. Genetic Modification of Neural Stem Cells. Molecular Therapy. 2008;16 3:450-457.

[97] Hu Z, Andang M, Ni D, Ulfendahl M. Neural cograft stimulates the survival and differentiation of embryonic stem cells in the adult mammalian auditory system. Brain Res. 2005;1051:137-144.

[98] Lang H, Schulte BA, Goddard JC, Hedrick M, Schulte JB, Wei L, et al. Transplantation of mouse embryonic stem cells into the cochlea of an auditory-neuropathy animal model: effects of timing after injury. J Assoc Res Otolaryngol. 2008;9:225-240.

[99] Corrales CE, Pan L, Li H, Liberman MC, Heller S, Edge AS. Engraftment and differentiation of embryonic stem cell-derived neural progenitor cells in the cochlear nerve trunk: growth of processes into the organ of Corti. J Neurobiol. 2006;66:1489-1500.

[100] Martinez-Monedero R, Corrales CE, Cuajungco MP, Heller S, Edge AS. Reinnervation of hair cells by auditory neurons after selective removal of spiral ganglion neurons. J Neurobiol. 2006; 66:319-331.

[101] Okano T, Nakagawa T, Endo T, Kim TS, Kita T, Tamura T, et al. Engraftment of embryonic stem cell-derived neurons into the cochlear modiolus. Neuroreport. 2005;16:1919-1922.

[102] Shi F, Corrales CE, Liberman MC, Edge AS. BMP4 induction of sensory neurons from human embryonic stem cells and reinnervation of sensory epithelium. Eur J Neurosci. 2007;26:3016-3023.

[103] Matsuoka AJ, Kondo T, Miyamoto RT, Hashino E. Enhanced survival of bone-marrow-derived pluripotent stem cells in an animal model of auditory neuropathy. The Laryngoscope. 2007;117:1629-1635.

[104] Hu Z, Ulfendahl M, Olivius NP. Central migration of neuronal tissue and embryonic stem cells following transplantation along the adult auditory nerve. Brain Res. 2004;1026:68-73.

[105] Ulfendahl M. Tissue transplantation into the inner ear. In: Martini A, Stephens D, Read A P. Genes, Hearing, and Deafness: From Molecular Biology to Clinical Practice. CRC Press. 2007. p. 294.

[106] Ito J, Murata M, Kawaguchi S. Regeneration and recovery of the hearing function of the central auditory pathway by transplants of embryonic brain tissue in adult rats. Exp Neurol. 2001;169:30-5.

[107] Lang H, Ebihara Y, Schmiedt RA, Minamiguchi H, Zhou D, Smythe N, et al. Contribution of bone marrow hematopoietic stem cells to adult mouse inner ear: mesenchymal cells and fibrocytes. J Comp Neurol. 2006;496: 187-201.

[108] Matsuoka AJ, Kondo T, Miyamoto RT, Hashino E. *In vivo* and *in vitro* characterization of bone marrow-derived stem cells in the cochlea. Laryngoscope. 2006;116:1363-1367.

[109] Chen W, Cacciabue-Rivolta DI, Moore HD, Rivolta MN. The human fetal cochlea can be a source for auditory progenitors/stem cells isolation. Hear Res. 2007;233:23-29.

[110] Nishimura K, Nakagawa T, Ito J. Potential of Pluripotent Stem Cells for the Replacement of Inner Ears, Embryonic Stem Cells - Recent Advances in Pluripotent Stem Cell-Based Regenerative Medicine, Prof. Craig Atwood editor. InTech. 2011; ISBN: 978-953-307-198-5, DOI: 10.5772/10541.

[111] Revoltella RP, Papini S, Rosellini A, et al. Cochlear repair by transplantation of human cord blood CD133+ cells to nod-scid mice made deaf with kanamycin and noise. Cell Transplant. 2008;17:665-78.

[112] Da Costa V, O'Grady G, Jackson L, Kaylie D, Raynor E. Improvements in sensorineural hearing loss after cord blood transplant in patients with mucopolysaccharidosis. Arch Otolaryngol Head Neck Surg. 2012;138:1071-6. DOI: 10.1001/jamaoto.2013.597.

[113] Available from: https://clinicaltrials.gov/show/NCT01343394 [Accessed: 2015-02-01].

[114] Forge A, Li L, Corwin JT, Nevill G. Ultrastructural evidence for hair cell regeneration in the mammalian inner ear. Sci. 1993;259:1616-1619.

[115] Warchol ME, Lambert PR, Goldstein BJ, Forge A, Corwin JT. Regenerative proliferation in inner ear sensory epithelia from adult guinea pigs and humans. Sci. 1993;259:1619-1622.

[116] Bauer PW, Geers AE, Brenner C, Moog JS, Smith RJH. The effect of GJB2 allele variants on performance after cochlear implantation. Laryngoscope. 2003;113:2135-41.

[117] Jane R Madell. Behavioral evaluation of hearing in infants and young children. New York : Thieme, 1998.

[118] Wright C, Burton H, Hall A, Moorthie S, Pokorska-Bocci A, et al. Next steps in the sequence. The implications of whole genome sequencing for health in the UK. Cambridge: 2011; PHG Foundation.

Chapter 5

Hearing Loss in Infectious and Contagious Diseases

Luiz Alberto Alves Mota, Paula Cristina Alves Leitão,
Paulo Marcelo Freitas de Barros and Ana Maria dos Anjos Carneiro Leão

Additional information is available at the end of the chapter

http://dx.doi.org/10.5772/61818

Abstract

Hearing loss can occur for various reasons, whether it is of a genetic, congenital or acquired character. Infectious diseases stand out among those causing this type of deficiency and account for approximately 25% of all cases of profound hearing loss. Of these, one-fifth are due to congenital causes. As to classifying hearing loss, this can be done according to where this is in the hearing system, to whether the loss is unilateral or bilateral, and to its intensity or degree. Regarding where the hearing system is affected, hearing loss can be about transmission (or conduction), perception (sensorineural), or mixed. Hearing losses arising from any affection of the outer and middle ear are called transmission or conductive losses. Sensorineural losses occur due to lesions on the hair cells of the cochlear organ of Corti (inner ear) and/or of the cochlear nerve. When there is concomitant conductive and sensorineural affection, the loss is classified as mixed. Hearing loss can interfere in the lives of affected individuals, since besides affecting communication, it can influence the quality of life, when the loss leads to feelings of sadness and anxiety, or even to social isolation. In children, it can moreover represent consequences for development. Thus, appropriate treatment and/or monitoring of infectious diseases is important, the purpose of which is to see to it that hearing loss is prevented or diagnosed early.

Keywords: Hearing loss, infectious diseases, etiology

1. Introduction

The hearing process begins when sound waves enter the outer ear and travel along the ear canal to the eardrum, causing it to vibrate. These vibrations are transmitted to the ossicles of the middle ear, which cause the sound vibration to be amplified before transmission to the inner ear. The inner ear has a part called the cochlea, which is filled with liquid and contains hair cells.[1]

The frequencies and intensities of the sound determine which hair cells will move. This causes electrical impulses to be generated and sent through the auditory pathways to the brain so that it may process the information. These electrical impulses are the codes that the brain can process and, on understanding them, assigns them various specific meanings.[1]

Hearing losses can be classified according to the location of the portion of the hearing system affected, to whether the loss is unilateral or bilateral, and to its intensity or degree. The location of the portion affected of hearing loss has to do with transmission (or conduction), perception (sensorineural), or a mixture of these (mixed). Sensorineural losses arising from some affection of the outer and middle ear are called transmission or conductive losses. Sensorineural losses result from lesions on the hair cells of the cochlear organ of Corti (inner ear) and/or of the cochlear nerve. When there are concomitant conductive and sensorineural affections, the hearing loss is classified as mixed.[2]

Hearing loss can occur due to a genetic, congenital, or acquired cause.[3] Among the acquired causes, many could sometimes be avoided, e.g., infections that occur during pregnancy, meningitis, and even due to using ototoxic medication.[4]

2. Epidemiology

Deafness is a global problem that affects individuals, families, societies, and governments. According to the World Health Organization (WHO), deafness affects between 1 and 4 people per 1,000 individuals, and there has been a considerable increase in poor countries. In 2005, for example, about 278 million people had degrees of hearing loss between moderate and profound, and 80% of them live in poor and developing countries.[5] Prevalence greater than 1 per 1000, however, indicates a serious public health problem that needs urgent attention.[6]

Infectious diseases are the leading cause of hearing loss and produce about 25% of profound losses. Of these, the causes of one-fifth are congenital.[7] The main infections include diseases such as rubella, cytomegalovirus, and measles.[7]

In the newborn, congenital infections are an important cause of hearing loss, which may have implications for the development of the child.[8]

3. Pathogenesis

The mechanisms that lead to the onset of viral hearing loss may include infections of the upper airways, may progress to subsequent involvement of the middle ear, and may occur with conductive hearing loss.[3]

Moreover, viral invasion of the inner ear can occur.[3] The viruses that can damage the inner ear may do so at different stages of the life cycle: during intrauterine life, childhood, adolescence, or adulthood. The pathological changes that predominate in the basal cochlea include degeneration of the organ of Corti, atrophy of the stria vascularis, displacement and distortion of the tectorial membrane, and degeneration of the saccule. The utricle and semicircular canals tend to be preserved.[9]

4. Main infectious and contagious diseases related to loss of hearing

4.1. Infections by virus

4.1.1. Epidemic parotiditis

Epidemic parotiditis or mumps is an acute systemic and contagious viral infection. A *Paramyxovirus*, with an RNA genome, is involved.[10]

The most typical clinical manifestations are sialadenitis, epididymo-orchitis, pancreatitis, meningitis, and hearing loss. Sensorineural hearing loss occurs in up to 5/10,000 cases and may appear some days or weeks after the parotiditis.[11]

Deafness is usually sudden, profound, associated with or without nausea, vomiting, dizziness, and tinnitus.[9] Hearing loss, which is unilateral in 80% of cases, is more common for high frequencies of sound and may present reduced caloric responses to the vestibular test.[11]

There may be atrophy of the organ of Corti and of the stria vascularis, with minimal effect on the vestibular system. Also observed are endolymphatic hydrops and obliteration of the endolymphatic duct.[11]

4.1.2. Infection by cytomegalovirus

Cytomegalovirus (CMV), which belongs to the herpesvirus family, is an enveloped virus that has the largest genome among the viruses that infect animal species. In immunocompetent individuals, it is generally responsible for asymptomatic infections.[12]

The highest incidence of the primary infection occurs in two peak periods: the first is in childhood, with early acquisition as a result of perinatal infection, and the second is in adolescence, through sexual transmission or by kissing.[12] It infects up to 70% of children who spend the day in kindergartens, and about 1–2% of infants are infected with CMV.[13]

In the congenital form, clinical manifestations range from the unapparent to the severe and widespread. Cytomegalic inclusion disease develops in about 5% of the infected fetuses. The most common manifestations at presentation are petechiae, hepatosplenomegaly, and jaundice. The occurrence of microcephaly with or without intracranial calcifications delayed intrauterine growth, and prematurity in 30–50% of cases is observed.[12] Deafness occurs in 20–65% of infants with this disease, which is typically bilateral.[13]

In patients with hearing loss, a consistent pattern follows, and this can develop over a period of years. Among asymptomatic patients, the rate of hearing loss of such children ranges from 7% to 13% and should therefore be considered in patients with nonsyndromic and nongenetic hearing loss.[13]

4.1.3. Rubella

This is a disease with an acute rash caused by an RNA virus of the genus *Rubivírus* and the Togaviridae family, which is highly contagious and mainly affects children.[13]

The clinical state is characterized by a maculopapular and diffuse pinpoint rash, starting on the face, scalp, and neck, later spreading to the trunk and limbs.[13]

The infection acquired after birth usually causes a mild or even subclinical disease. The main symptoms of this form are retroauricular, cervical and suboccipital lymphadenopathy, rash, and fever. Complications are uncommon.[10]

Maternal infection during early pregnancy can lead to infection of the fetus, resulting in congenital rubella.[10] Congenital rubella syndrome (Gregg's syndrome) affects most organ systems, causing cataracts, microphthalmia, heart defects, skin rash, retardation of growth, and hearing loss. In general, hearing loss affects about 50% of individuals with the disease and is normally severe to profound. Auditory manifestations may occur months to years after the initial infection.[11]

4.1.4. Measles

Measles is an acutely infectious viral disease that is potentially serious, transmittable, and extremely contagious. Its etiologic agent is an RNA virus of the genus *Morbillivirus*, family Paramyxoviridae.[13]

Among the clinical manifestations, it is characterized by high fever, above 38.5°C, a widespread maculopapular rash, cough, coryza, conjunctivitis, and Koplik spots (small white spots on the oral mucosa, prior to the rash).[13]

It may cause severe degeneration of the organ of Corti, the stria vascularis, cochlear neurons, and vestibular damage. Inflammation, fibrous deposit, and ossification in the basal turn of the cochlea may also be present. Hearing loss tends to be asymmetrical, bilateral, and severe. Vestibular abnormalities are not rare.[11]

4.1.5. Viral meningitis

Viral meningitis is characterized by a clinical state of neurological changes, which usually develops benignly. Approximately 85% of cases are due to the group of Enteroviruses, among which the poliovirus, echovirus, and coxsackievirus stand out. Other less common groups are arboviruses, herpes simplex virus, and varicella, mumps, and measles viruses.[14]

It occurs most frequently in children over two years old and can lead to sensorineural hearing loss.[3]

4.1.6. Herpes simplex

Herpes simplex has been considered one of the most common viral contamination agents in humans and is subdivided into two groups: type 1 and type 2.[15]

Infections caused by herpes simplex type 1 usually affect areas such as the lips, mouth, intraoral region, nose, eyes, while infections caused by herpes simplex type 2 are mainly found in the genital and surrounding areas. Trigger factors include fever, exposure to cold temperatures or ultraviolet rays, skin or mucous abrasions, emotional stress, and nerve injury. In the case of occurrence in newborns, the onset of infection can be at different periods: prenatal (congenital infection), perinatal (infection through the birth canal), or postnatal (infection through contact with infected individuals).[15]

The virus of the herpes group is regarded as causing sensorineural loss. In pregnancy, it can also cause spontaneous miscarriages, still births, and congenital defects.[15]

4.1.7. Infectious mononucleosis and other viral agents

Infectious mononucleosis (IM) is caused by the Epstein–Barr virus (EBV), characterized by fever, pharyngitis, lymphadenopathy, and atypical lymphocytosis. EBV is a member of the Herpesviridae family.

One of the main viral agents associated with sensorineural hearing loss in adulthood is the IM virus. Other agents that can also often affect this age-group and are related to hearing loss are adenovirus, enterovirus, influenza, and parainfluenza.[3]

4.2. Infections by bacteria

4.2.1. Bacterial meningitis

Meningitis is frequently associated with a high mortality rate. A large portion may still present sequelae of the disease, among which is hearing loss. This disease is held to be among the main ones responsible for postnatal acquired hearing impairment.[16]

Among the mechanisms elucidated, as being responsible for hearing damage, is the direct invasion of the bacteria into the cochlea and labyrinth, lesion of cranial nerve VIII, by toxins, and blockage of small vessels and ototoxic action of the antibiotics used. Regarding the degree of loss, a high percentage of profound hearing loss (66.95%) has been evidenced. However, hearing loss of all degrees (mild to anacusis) was observed.[16]

In a study of 124 children recruited from 21 hospitals in England and South Wales, aged between 4 weeks and 16 years old, with a recent diagnosis of bacterial meningitis, 92 (74%) had meningococcal and 18 (15%) had pneumococcal meningitis. All cases showed obvious hearing loss in the first assessment. Three children had permanent sensorineural hearing loss. Thirteen children (10.5%) had reversible loss, nine of which were resolved within 48 hours of diagnosis.[17]

The impact on the development of the child after meningitis can be devastating. In the postmeningitis period, a possibility of rehabilitation for patients with severe and profound sensorineural loss is a cochlear implant.[18]

In cases of postmeningitis hearing loss, it is particularly important to do the implant as early as possible due to the intracochlear ossification that may occur, thus preventing the placement of electrodes in the lumen of the cochlea.[19]

4.2.2. Syphilis

During the decade of 2003–2012, the diagnosis of primary syphilis increased 61% in men in England, while in contrast, this diagnosis in women decreased by 16%.[20] In the 2004 Sentinela Parturiente (Mother in Labour Sentinel) Study of the Ministry of Health in Brazil, the prevalence of syphilis in pregnant women was 1.6%, about four times higher than HIV infection in the same group, the estimate being that a total of 48,425 pregnant women were infected in that year. Between 2005 and June 2012, 57,700 cases of syphilis in pregnant women were registered in SINAN (the Brazilian statutory body for notifiable diseases), most of which occurred in the Southeast and Northeast regions.[21]

Syphilis is an infectious disease caused by a bacterium, *Treponema pallidum,* which is predominantly transmitted sexually. If left untreated, the disease can progress to stages that adversely affect the skin and internal organs such as the heart, liver, and nervous system central.[18] Hearing loss can occur because of syphilis, but currently this is rare, and this being most often in the tertiary phase.[3]

Otosyphilis may be present in the form of a sudden and fluctuating sensorineural loss, episodic vertigo, with progressive unilateral or bilateral loss.[11]

Acquired syphilis may also affect the inner ear, simulating Ménière's disease. Hearing loss can progress rapidly progressive, initially with good discrimination; tinnitus and vestibular symptoms disappear to the extent that the destruction of the labyrinth is completed.[9]

Congenital syphilis is due to the hematogenous spread of *Treponema pallidum* of pregnant women who have not been treated or inadequately treated for their unborn child, via the placenta. Transmission can occur at any stage of pregnancy and in any stage of the disease.[22]

Congenital syphilis can cause severe deafness and separately affect both ears. Manifestation occurs when a child is around two years old or between 8 and 20 years old.[9]

4.3. Protozoan infections

4.3.1. Toxoplasmosis

Toxoplasmosis is caused by infection with the obligate intracellular parasite *Toxoplasma gondii.* Both in its acute and in its chronic form, it is related to the appearance of a clinically evident disease, including lymphadenopathy, encephalitis, myocarditis, and pneumonitis.[10]

In immunocompetent individuals, acute toxoplasmosis is habitually asymptomatic and goes unnoticed in 80–90% of adults and children with acquired infection. In the congenital form, the infection of the placenta determines the hematogenous infection of the fetus. The proportion of fetuses that are infected increases as pregnancy progresses, but the severity of the infection declines.[10]

Toxoplasma gondii has been associated with lesion of the auditory pathways with a demonstration of calcium deposits (similar to the calcifications found in the brains of children with congenital toxoplasmosis) in the spiral ligament and the cochlea. A hearing deficit has been reported in about 20% of cases of congenital toxoplasmosis.[23]

5. Final remarks

Hearing loss can interfere with the life of affected individuals because in addition to affecting communication, this can influence the quality of life, on expressing feelings such as sadness and anxiety, or can even lead to social isolation. In infancy, hearing loss can still represent consequences for development.

Thus, proper treatment and/or monitoring of infectious diseases for the purpose of establishing the prevention or early diagnosis of hearing loss is important. With regard to congenital infections, public measures that encourage primary prevention and early identification of these affections in newborns are needed. Therefore, hearing health will depend on epidemiological studies of each location and on a perfect integration between health and education authorities working in an integrated way with all other sectors of society.

Author details

Luiz Alberto Alves Mota[1*], Paula Cristina Alves Leitão[2], Paulo Marcelo Freitas de Barros[3] and Ana Maria dos Anjos Carneiro Leão[4]

*Address all correspondence to: luizmota10@hotmail.com

1 Faculty of Medical Sciences, Universidade de Pernambuco, Brazil

2 Faculty of Medical Sciences, Universidade de Pernambuco, Recife/PE, Brazil

3 Universidade Católica de Pernambuco, Brazil

4 Department of Animal Morphology and Physiology, Universidade Federal Rural de Pernambuco, Brazil

References

[1] Instituto Brasileiro do sono. Available at: http://www.institutobrasileirodosono.com.br/. Accessed on 16 November 2014.

[2] Vieira ABC, Macedo LR, Gonçalves DU. O diagnóstico da perda auditiva na infância. Pediatria (São Paulo). 2007; 29(1):43–49.

[3] Vieira ABC, Mancini P, Goncalves DU. Infectious diseases and hearing loss. Rev Med Minas Gerais. 2010; 20(1): 102–6.

[4] Pereira T, Costa KC, Pomilio MCA, Costa SMS, Rodrigues GRI, Sartorato EL. Investigação etiológica da deficiência auditiva em neonatos identificados em um programa de triagem auditiva neonatal universal. Rev. CEFAC. 2014; 16(2): 422–9.

[5] World Health Organization. Deafness and hearing impairment. Available at: http://www.who.int/mediacentre/factsheets/fs300/en/index.html. Accessed on 21 January 2010.

[6] Bubbico, LRA.; Spagnolo, A. Prevalence of prelingual deafness in Italy. Acta Otorhinolaryngol. 2007; 27: 17–21.

[7] Catlin FI. Prevention of hearing impairment from infection and ototoxic drugs. Arch Otolaryngol. 1985; 111(6):377–84.

[8] Gatto CI, Tochetto TM. Infantile hearing loss: implications and solutions. Rev CEFAC. 2007; 9(1): 110–15.

[9] Miniti, Aroldo. Otorrinolaringologia: Clínica e Cirúrgica. 2a edição. São Paulo: Editora Atheneu, 2000.

[10] Harrison. Medicina interna. 17º edição. Rio de Janeiro: McGraw-Hill Interamericana do Brasil, 2008.

[11] K. J. Lee. Princípios de Otorrinolaringologia. Cirurgia cabeça e pescoço. 9º edição. São Paulo: McGraw-Hill, 2008.

[12] Mendrone Junior, A. Prevalência da infecção pelo citomegalovírus: a importância de estudos locais. Rev Bras Hematol Hemoter. 2010; 32(1): 7–8.

[13] Brasil. Ministério da Saúde. Secretaria de Vigilância em Saúde. Guia de Vigilância em Saúd. Brasília: Ministério da Saúde, 2014. Available at: <www.saude.gov.br/bvs> Accessed on 13 February 2015.

[14] Secretaria de Estado da Saúde de São Paulo. Divisão de Doenças de Transmissão Respiratória. Meningites virais. Rev Saúde Pública. 2006; 40(4), 748–50.

[15] Schuster LC, Buss C. Herpes and its hearing implications: a literature review. Rev. CEFAC. 2009; 11(4):695–700.

[16] Romero, JH., Carvalho, MS., Feniman, MR. Achados audiológicos em indivíduos pós-meningite. Rev Saúde Pública. 1997; 31(4): 398–401.

[17] Richardson MP, Reid A, Tarlow MJ, Rudd PT. Hearing loss during bacterial meningitis. Arch Dis Child. 1997; 76:134–8.

[18] Bevilacqua MC, Moret ALM, Costa Filho OA, Nascimento LT, Banhara MR. Cochlear implant in deaf children due to meningitis. Rev Bras Otorhinolaryngol. 2003; 69(6): 760–4.

[19] Implante coclear. Available at: http://www.forl.org.br/pdf/seminarios/seminario_1.pdf. Accessed on 15 February 2015.

[20] Recent epidemiology of infectious syphilis and congenital syphilis. Available at: https://www.gov.uk/government/publications/infectious-syphilis-and-congenital-syphilis-recent-epidemiology. Accessed on 10 April 2015.

[21] Boletim epidemiológico sífilis 2012. Situação epidemiológica da sífilis no Brasil—1998–2012. Ministério da saúde, 2012. Available at: http://bvsms.saude.gov.br/bvs/periodicos/boletim_epidem_sifilis_2012.pdf. Accessed on 10 April 2015.

[22] Secretaria de Estado da Saúde SES-SP. Sífilis congênita e sífilis na gestação. Rev. Saúde Pública. 2008; 42 (4): 768–72.

[23] Andrade GMQ, Resende LM, Goulart EMA, Siqueira AL, Vitor RWA, Januario JN. Deficiência auditiva na toxoplasmose congênita detectada pela triagem neonatal. Rev Bras Otorhinolaryngol. 2008; 74(1):21–8.

Section 2

Hearing Loss and the Voice

Chapter 6

Hearing Loss and the Voice

Ana Cristina Coelho, Daniela Malta Medved and
Alcione Ghedini Brasolotto

Additional information is available at the end of the chapter

http://dx.doi.org/10.5772/61217

Abstract

The voice varies according to the context of speech and to the physical and psychological conditions of the human being, and there is always a normal standard for the vocal output. Hearing loss can impair voce production, causing social, educational, and speech limitations, with specific deviation of the communication related to speech and voice. Usually, the voice is not the main focus of the speech-language pathology therapy with individuals with hearing loss, but its deviations can represent such a negative impact on this population that it can interfere on speech intelligibility and crucially compromise the social integration of the individual. The literature vastly explores acoustic and perceptual characteristics of children and adults with hearing loss. Voice problems in individuals with this impairment are directly related to its type and severity, age, gender, and type of hearing device used. While individuals with mild and moderate hearing loss can only present problems with resonance, severely impaired individuals may lack intensity and frequency control, among other alterations. The commonly found vocal deviations include strain, breathiness, roughness, monotone, absence of rhythm, unpleasant quality, hoarseness, vocal fatigue, high pitch, reduced volume, loudness with excessive variation, unbalanced resonance, altered breathing pattern, brusque vocal attack, and imprecise articulation. These characteristics are justified by the incapability of the deaf to control their vocal performance due to the lack of auditory monitoring of their own voice, caused by the hearing loss. Hence, the development of an intelligible speech with a good quality of voice on the hearing impaired is a challenge, despite the sophisticated technological advances of hearing aids, cochlear implants and other implantable devices. The purpose of this chapter is therefore to present an extensive review of the literature and describe our experience regarding the evaluation, diagnosis, and treatment of voice disorders in individuals with hearing loss.

Keywords: Hearing loss, voice, voice quality

1. Introduction

Didactically, the voice is described as the resulting sound of the vibration of the vocal folds, which is amplified by the vocal tract resonators. The vocal tract articulators modify this sound producing recognizable vowels and consonants. A pleasant and socially acceptable voice production is highly dependent on emotional, social, and physical conditions, the latter including auditory monitoring of the voice.

Hearing loss can impair oral communication, causing social, educational, and speech limitations, with specific deviation of the communication related to speech and voice. Usually, the rehabilitation process prioritizes auditory abilities, and therefore, the voice is not the main focus of the speech-language therapy with individuals with hearing loss. Its deviations, however, can represent such a negative impact on this population that it can interfere on speech intelligibility, cause a negative impact on the listener, and crucially compromise the social integration of the individual.

The challenges of voice production in individuals with hearing loss involve alterations in respiration, phonation, and articulation [1]. Also, voice problems in individuals with this impairment are directly related to its type and severity, age, gender, and type of hearing device used [2]. While individuals with mild and moderate hearing loss can only present problems with resonance, severely impaired individuals may lack intensity and frequency control, among other alterations [3]. Hence, the development of an intelligible speech with a good quality of voice in individuals with hearing loss is a challenge, despite the sophisticated technological advances of hearing aids, cochlear implants and other implantable devices.

2. The auditory system and voice production

Voice production (Figures 1A–1H) occurs by the integration of the respiratory, phonatory and articulatory systems, and also involves highly complex mechanisms of structures related to the central and peripheral nervous systems (Figure 1A) [4]. The airflow that is moved out of the lungs during expiration by the coordinated action of the diaphragm, abdominal muscles, chest muscles, and rib cage is directed toward the vocal folds (Figure 1B). Then to produce sound, the vocal folds are moved to midline by the action intrinsic muscles, nerves, and cartilages (Figures 1B–1D). The column of air from the lungs creates subglottic pleasure, causing the opening of the vocal folds. This is the beginning of a vibratory cycle that occurs repeatedly. In one vibratory cycle, the column of air pressure opens the bottom of the vocal folds. Then the air continues to move upward, now toward the top of the vocal folds, opening them entirely. The low pressure created behind the fast-moving air column produces the "Bernoulli effect", which causes the bottom to close, followed by the top. The closure of the vocal folds cuts off the air column and releases a pulse of air, and the cycle recommences (Figure 1E). The rapid pulses of air created in the repeated vibratory cycles produce "voiced sounds", which is then amplified and modified by the vocal tract resonators. The nose, pharynx, and mouth amplify and modify sound, allowing it to take on the distinctive qualities of voice. Finally, the articulators produce recognizable words [5] (Figures 1F–1G).

The neural component of the voice production generates two components for the voice: a propositional and an emotional one. The propositional vocalization is the expression of any idea that can be an abstract thought, an action, or an appreciation. Its content is not important if it has a communication proposal by means of the voice. The emotional vocalization expresses the emotional components of phonation. Both systems converge or integrate in the brainstem region where the retroambiguus nuclei are located. There, a new recording and a new result occur. This information goes to the nucleus ambiguus and retrofacial nucleus, which originate the vagal fibers of superior and inferior (recurrent) laryngeal nerves [6]. The peripheral nerves directly related the voice, providing sensory and motor innervation of the vocal tract include the glossopharyngeal nerve (IX cranial nerve), the trigeminal nerve (V cranial nerve), the facial nerve (VII cranial nerve), the vagus nerve (X cranial nerve), and the hypoglossal nerve (XII cranial nerve) [6].

Voice and speech production is therefore a complex process and involves numerous regulatory mechanisms [7]. In addition, during the whole process of maturation of the voice, people develop phonatory control and abilities to regulate and vary the voice use in different situations, which is directly related to a key component, which is the auditory feedback of the voice [8].

The auditory system is essential to regulate voice production by monitoring different voice parameters [9]. It provides two types of control over speech production: feedback control and feedforward control [10]. The feedback control monitors task performance during execution and also deviations from the desired performance, which are corrected according to sensory information. In the feedforward control, task performance is executed from previously learned commands, without reliance on incoming task-related sensory information. Speech and voice production involve both feedforward and feedback control, and auditory feedback impacts both control processes [11] (Figure 2).

Also, the auditory system has three roles: providing information regarding voice targets, which is important for corrections in pitch, volume, and other attributes that may affect intelligibility of speech; providing feedback about environmental conditions, which is important in noisy situations, for example, so that the speaker knows to enunciate more clearly, to increase amplitude, and to reduce speaking rate to increase intelligibility; and contributing to the generation of internal models for the motor plans for voice production, which is essential to the maintenance of a rapid speech rate through development of internal models, allowing for the vocal tract and related structures to be prepared before vocalization and for speech to continue without constant auditory feedback [10, 12]. These roles are responsible, therefore, for modeling voice quality, pitch, loudness, resonance, articulation, and speech rate.

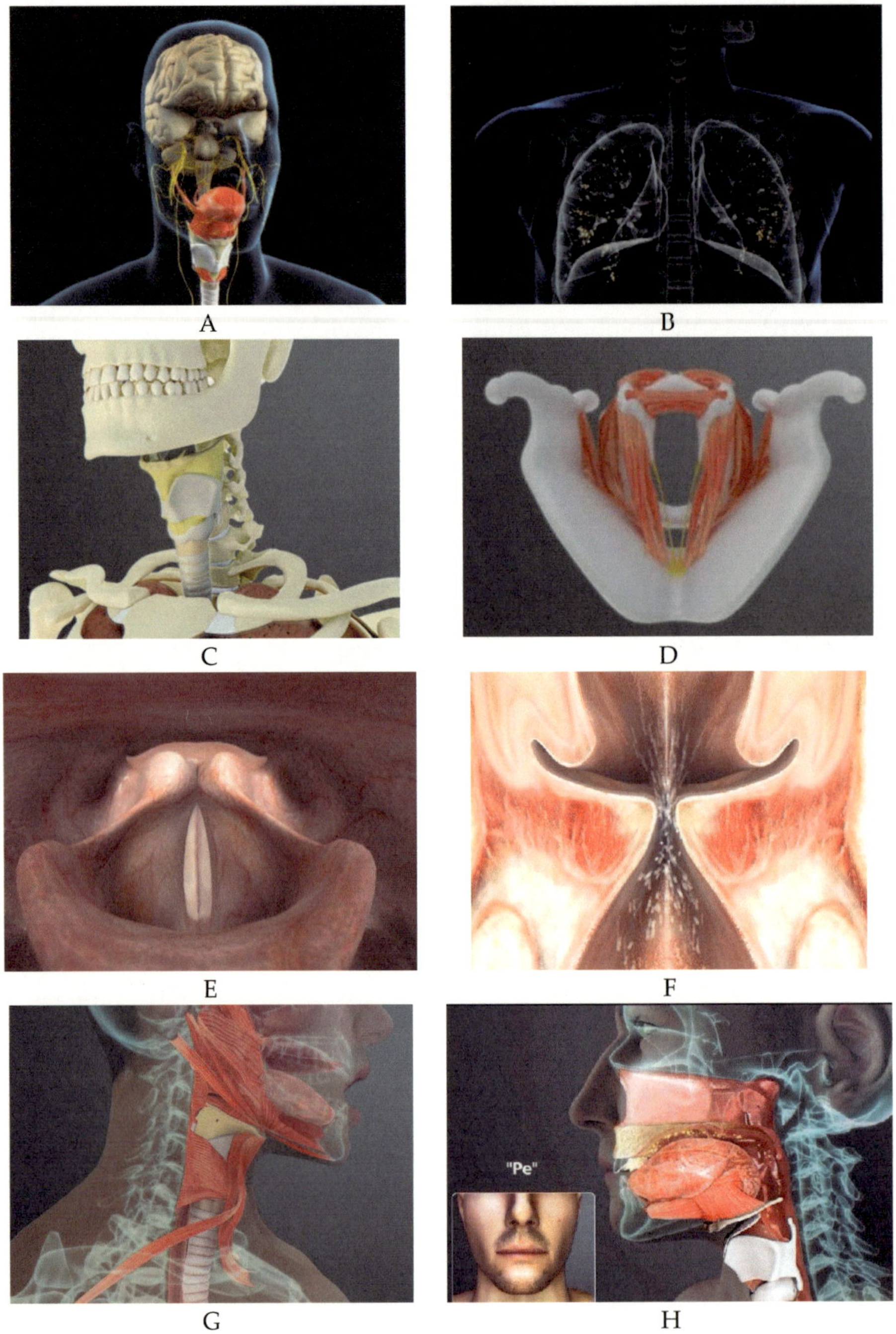

Figure 1. Voice production. (A) Peripheral innervation of the vocal tract; (B) respiration; (C) larynx; (D) intrinsic muscles of the larynx; (E) vibratory cycle; (F) vocal fold adduction; (G) extrinsic muscles of the larynx; (H) resonators and articulators. Source: Virtual Man Project [4].

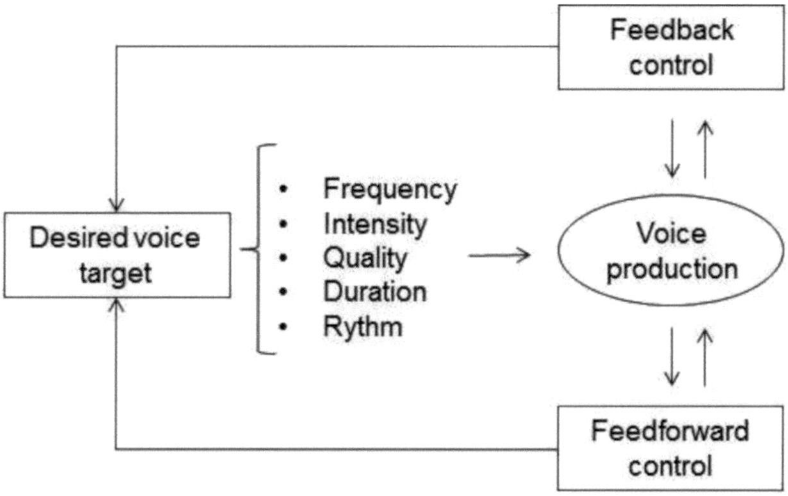

Figure 2. Auditory monitoring of voice production.

3. The voice of individuals with hearing loss

The overall product of a deaf speaker's vocal apparatus depends on the respiratory conditions, laryngeal state, resonators, articulators and prosodic aspects such as intensity, intonation, rhythm, and frequency.

Respiration aspects related to phonation can also be altered in this population. Laryngeal aerodynamics between children with bilateral profound sensorineural hearing loss using hearing aids and normal hearing children were compared by measuring vital capacity, peak flow, maximum sustained phonation, and fast abduction-adduction rate [13]. The authors found significant differences between vital capacity, maximum sustained phonation, and abduction-adduction rate, but not air flow, suggesting the presence of physiologically healthy and functional lungs for the airflow supply that will be required for speech production, but a limited use of the lung volume, poor management of the air supply, and poor laryngeal control during phonation.

Another potential factor that affects voice and speech intelligibility in individuals with hearing loss is the articulation accuracy of consonants and vowels. It is important to consider that voice and articulation are closely related since the sound that comes from the larynx is transformed into words by its combination with the dynamic and static structures of the upper vocal tract.

The phonetic inventory of the consonants in individuals with hearing loss can be compromised by distortions, substitutions, and omissions. Some phonological processes such as deletion of final consonants, cluster reduction, stopping, and devoicing may also occur [14], especially with voiced sounds and high frequency fricative consonants. The articulation of individuals with hearing loss has been reported to be characterized by the absence of some fricatives, the presence of distortions, and phonological disorders [15]. An adequate vowel production depends on the shape of the lips and position of the tongue and is also affected by the lack of auditory monitoring of the voice [16].

Regarding all aspects of voice production, the voice of individuals with hearing loss has been widely described. Specifically, acoustic and perceptual findings (Tables 1 and 2) indicate alterations that go from minor loudness deviation to significant respiratory, phonatory, and articulatory disorders. However, these characteristics are inconsistent and not unanimous among authors. They are reported to depend on age of hearing loss onset, its type and severity, and on the treatment of choice (Table 1) and have been compared among groups of patients in different conditions: prelingually deafened and postlingually deafened, aided and unaided, pre and post cochlear implantation, and patients treated with either hearing aids or cochlear implants (Table 2).

Such a variety of vocal features and results (Tables 1 and 2) are possibly due different methodological approaches with different assessment conditions, such as different speech materials, different assessment techniques, different software, different perceptual protocols, number of participants, different age range, different hearing devices, different age at the activation of the hearing device, and presence or absence of a control group to establish normative data [17]. Therefore, the understanding of speech and voice production of individuals with hearing loss is still a challenge and is missing a standardized approach.

	HL characteristics	Voice characteristics
Type	Conductive	Reduced loudness [3]
	Sensorineural	High fundamental frequency (f_0) [18–21], f_0 within normal standards [15], normal jitter [15], normal shimmer [15], high variation of amplitude, and f_0 [22] instability [23,24]
	Mixed	Not reported
Severity	Mild to moderate	Resonance disorder [3]
	Severe to profound	High f_0 [18,25,26], instability [23,24,26,27]
Hearing loss onset	Prelingual	Hoarseness [28], breathiness [28], strain [26,28], high f_0 [20,25,26], high variability in f_0 [21,26], excessive intonation [21], monotone [20], excessive pitch variation [21], altered speech rate [21], increased loudness [21,29], loudness either to soft or too loud [20], resonance irregularity [17,21,30], instability [24,26]
	Postlingual	Abnormal intonation [21,28], high pitch/f_0 [21,31], altered speech rate [21,28], nasality [2,21], loudness deviation [2,21,28,31], roughness [1], strain [1], instability [1], high jitter [31], high shimmer [31] high noise to harmonic ratio [31]
Treatment	Hearing aid	High f_0 [19,32], high pitch [10], f_0 within normal standards [22], normal jitter [22], normal shimmer [22], high jitter [32], high shimmer [32], high variation of amplitude and f_0 [22], strain [17], instability [17, 30]

	HL characteristics	Voice characteristics
	Cochlear implant	High f_0 [19,26,33], normal f_0 [24,34], high pitch [17,26], variation of amplitude and fundamental frequency [22], high jitter and shimmer [32,33], instability [17,23,24,26], strain [10,19], significant overall severity of voice quality [26,35]

Table 1. Voice characteristic of individuals with hearing loss according to type and severity of hearing loss, hearing loss onset, and treatment of choice.

Comparison	Title	Results
Hearing loss onset	Acoustic analysis of the voice in pediatric cochlear implant recipients: a longitudinal study [19]	Normalization of the long-term amplitude control after cochlear implantation regardless of onset
	Acoustic analysis of voice in cochlear implant recipients with postmeningitic hearing loss [36]	No significant differences found regarding hearing loss onset
Unaided individuals × normal hearing adults	Acoustic features of voice in patients with severe hearing loss [31]	Deviated acoustic parameters for the unaided participants
Pre- to post cochlear implantation	Voice analysis of postlingually deaf adults pre- and post-cochlear implantation [1]	Improved overall severity, strain, loudness, and instability with cochlear implantation as well as reduction in fundamental frequency and its variability
	Change of phonation control after cochlear implantation [20]	Decrease of jitter, shimmer, fundamental frequency and amplitude variability in prelingually deafened children, and no significant differences in postlingually deafened adults. Even so, the children's voices were worse than the adults'
	Effect of cochlear implantation on nasality in children [27]	Significant reduction of nasality after cochlear implantation
Hearing aid × cochlear implant	Comparison of the overall intelligibility, articulation, resonance, and voice characteristics between children using cochlear implants and those using bilateral hearing aids: a pilot study [37]	Better intelligibility for users of cochlear implants and no differences in the remaining parameters
Cochlear implant × hearing aid × normal hearing	Objective voice quality in children using cochlear implants: a multiparameter approach [17]	Both groups with hearing loss presented with altered perceptual scores, with worse results for the

Comparison	Title	Results
		hearing aided children; no significant differences in acoustic measures were observed
	The influence of the auditory prosthesis type on deaf children's voice quality [32]	Better results for the participants with hearing aids
	Acoustic, aerodynamic, and perceptual analyses of the voice of cochlear-implanted children [35]	Better voice quality for children with cochlear implants
	Voice and pronunciation of cochlear implant speakers [38]	Better results for the participants with cochlear implants
Cochlear implant × normal hearing	Cochlear implanted children present voice parameters within normal standards [24]	Higher instability and frequency variation for cochlear implant users.
	An initial study of voice characteristics of children using two different sound coding strategies in comparison to normal hearing children [26]	Higher fundamental frequency, fundamental frequency variability, amplitude variability, overall severity, strain, loudness, instability, high pitch, and resonance deviation for the cochlear implanted participants
	Nasalance and nasality in children with cochlear implants and children with hearing aids [30]	Children with hearing aids and cochlear implants showed altered nasalance. Cul-de-sac resonance was observed on a significantly larger scale than in the normal hearing group, and children with were significantly more hypernasal in than normal hearing children
	Normal-like motor speech parameters measured in children with long-term cochlear implant experience using a novel objective analytic technique [39]	Cochlear implant users had poorer than normal intonation stimulability, particularly frequency variability
Hearing aid × normal hearing	Laryngeal aerodynamics in children with hearing impairment versus age- and height-matched normal hearing peers [13]	Significant difference in the vital capacity, maximum sustained phonation, and fast adduction abduction rate
	Variability in voice fundamental frequency of sustained vowels in	Significantly higher low frequency modulation for the individuals with hearing loss

Comparison	Title	Results
	speakers with sensorineural hearing loss [40]	
	Voice field measurements–a new method of examination: the influence of hearing on the human voice [41]	Voice field of the impaired person is significantly limited in regard to both frequency and dynamics, and it is narrower than that of intact persons.

Table 2. Overview of findings of voice characteristics when comparing hearing loss onset, treatment, and normal hearing.

3.1. Perceptual ratings of the voice of individuals with hearing loss

The auditory-perceptual evaluation of the voice is a key element to understand the voice production of individuals with hearing loss. When associated with acoustics, aerodynamics, laryngeal imaging, and quality of life, it gives a complete background to define the best treatment approach. Although it is subjective and depends on listener's experience, the auditory perception is the main upholder of voice therapy, and it can be correlated to all of the assessments cited.

The voice of the individuals with hearing loss has been perceptively characterized using several scales: the Voice Profile Analysis [42], the GRBAS scale [43], the GRBASI scale [44], the Prosody-Voice Screening Profile (PVSP) [45], the Consensus Auditory-Perceptual Evaluation of Voice (CAPE-V) [46], and visual analog scales of specific parameters [47]. Theses scales 14 can be used to characterize voice quality and quantify the vocal alteration.

Reported characteristics in the last 10 years include significant overall severity of dysphonia [17, 26, 35, 48], roughness [17], strain [17, 16, 48], resonance deviations [26, 48], high pitch [1, 26], and instability [24, 26].

One particular study [21], described the voice characteristics of 40 profoundly hearing-impaired young adults using the Voice Profile Analysis (VPA), which includes articulatory (supralaryngeal) settings, laryngeal settings, strain, and prosodic settings of the voice tract. The comparison with a control group showed some interesting data for the individuals with hearing loss:

- Range of movements: minimized tongue movements, both minimized and extensive jaw movement, and both minimized and extensive lip movements
- Pitch and loudness: narrow pitch range, low pitch variability, low loudness mean, narrow loudness range, and low loudness variability
- Tension: pharyngeal constriction, both laryngeal tension and looseness
- Laryngeal factors: harshness, use of falsetto, raised larynx

Considering these findings, the positioning, movement, and strain of the articulatory organs seem worthy of further study as they shape the voice tract and determine some aspects of voice quality.

In terms of resonance, the most reported characteristic in individuals with hearing loss is nasality. The abnormal nasalization of vowels and nasal consonants significantly contributes to the abnormal voicing of children and adults with hearing loss, which is related to poor control of the velopharyngeal valve due to the lack of auditory feedback–oral/nasal distinctions [28] and is related to the duration if the hearing impairment [2] and speech rate [27]. The velopharyngeal valve lack rhythm and strength in this population, despite normal structure and muscle activity [49].

A mixed resonance, however, is not an uncommon feature. A pharyngeal resonance also known as cul-de-sac [30, 50] can also be found and is associated with elevation of the hyoid and retraction of the tongue [51]. Hyponasality is also reported [52]. Thirty profoundly deaf children [42] had significantly higher nasalance values compared with a normal hearing control group when nasal consonants were absent (reflecting hypernasality) and significantly lower when an utterance was loaded heavily with nasal consonants (reflecting hyponasality).

The suprasegmental features of speech that are conveyed by the parameters of fundamental frequency, intensity, and duration can directly affect the voice production and speech intelligibility. These features constitute prosody, which is considered the "melody and rhythm of spoken language" [53]. During the development of oral communication, how children acquire target appropriate prosodic structure is important because it plays a role in many aspects of linguistic function, from lexical stress to grammatical structure to emotional effect. It is therefore important for the transmission of meaning and thus for intelligibility. These aspects of the oral communication can be problematic for individuals with hearing loss since auditory monitoring is critical for listeners' recognition of prosodic contrasts of speech [54]. An investigation of the production of speech intonation in cochlear implanted children in comparison with their age-matched peers with normal hearing [54] found inappropriate intonation contours for the implanted participants. Another study found that cochlear implanted children present restriction of intonation, particularly in interrogative sentences [55].

3.2. Acoustic characteristics

The acoustic analysis is an instrumental assessment that complements the auditory perceptive evaluation and provides quantitative and qualitative information about voice behavior from the analysis of the sound signal. By using computerized software, it is possible to obtain measures of fundamental frequency, perturbation and noise indexes, temporal changes in speech, and also visual graphic interpretation. This assessment magnifies the understanding of voice behavior and allows the documentation of treatment outcome.

The voice characteristics of the individual with hearing loss can be visually measured or numerically evidenced in the acoustic analysis and depend on the anatomy and physiology of the entire vocal tract. For example, the fundamental frequency can be influenced by the length, elongation, mass, and tension of the vocal folds and is integrated with the subglottic pressure. The higher fundamental frequency observed in individuals with hearing loss is related to greater tension during voice production as a result of the search for kinesthetic monitoring [41].

Also, individuals with hearing loss have difficulties in maintaining the stability of the fundamental frequency [56], during the extension of a vowel and during connected speech.

In Figure 3, the emissions of the sustained /a/ vowel by two men with 27 years of age, one with hearing loss and one with normal hearing, are presented. It is possible to visualize the greater instability in frequency (blue) and intensity (gray) and also higher fundamental frequency (203 Hz) produced by the individual with hearing loss in comparison to the individual with normal hearing (87Hz).

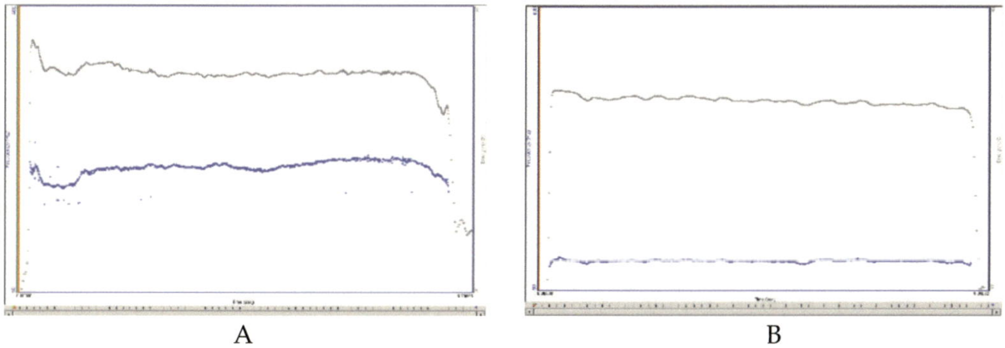

Figure 3. Graphs with fundamental frequency (blue) and intensity (gray) of the voices of an individual with hearing loss (A) and an individual with normal hearing (B) during the emission of a sustained vowel, obtained with the program Real Time Pitch from KayPentax.

Figure 4 shows the excessive variation of frequency of a child with 4 years of age with hearing loss in comparison to a child with the same age and with normal hearing while counting numbers.

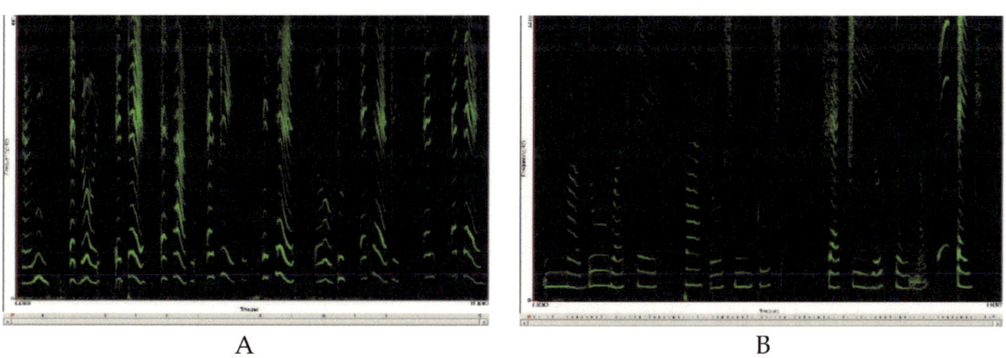

Figure 4. Graphs with spectrograms of the sequential speech of a child with hearing loss and a child with normal hearing, obtained with the Multi Speech software from KayPentax.

The acoustic evaluation can be performed visually by describing the spectrogram, a tridimensional graph the present the following information obtained by the Fourier transformation:

the frequency in the ordinate axis, measured in Hertz; the time in the abscissa axis, measured in seconds; and the intensity, according to the degree of darkening or coloration of the spectrum, measured in decibel [57].

Figure 5 shows the spectrograms of a woman with 32 years of age with hearing loss and of another with the same age and normal hearing, evidencing greater irregularity of the sustentation of the emission, greater presence of noise, greater spacing between the harmonics, intensity, and effort in the voice of the woman with hearing loss.

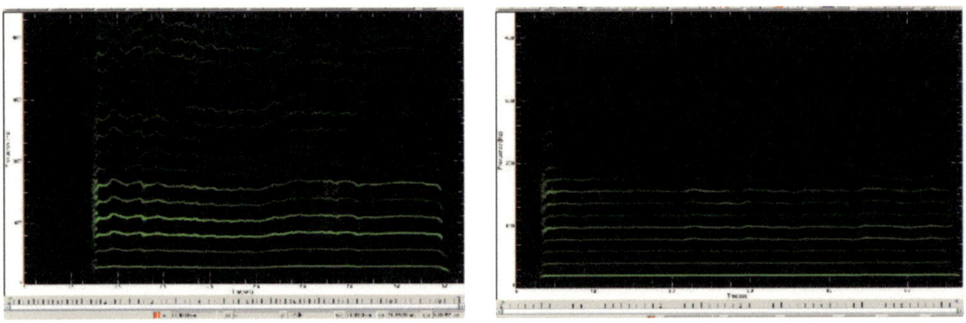

A B

Figure 5. Graphs with spectrograms of the sustained vowel of a woman with hearing loss (A) and a woman with normal hearing (B) obtained with the Multi Speech program from KayPentax.

Some perturbations of the sound wave and of the ratio of noise in relation to the harmonics were used by some authors to characterize the voice of individuals with hearing loss. These characteristics can be related to the perception of roughness and strain in the voice. Generally, the voices of individuals with hearing loss show more perturbation of the sound wave and greater quantity of noise in relation to individuals with normal hearing [58]. Among the measures of perturbation, the jitter indicates short-term variability of the fundamental frequency. These values can represent a small variation in mass or tension of the vocal folds, on the distribution of mucus on them, on the symmetry of the structures, or even in the muscular or neural activity involved; the shimmer indicates short-term variability of the amplitude of the sound wave, and it is a measure of phonatory stability. Its values increase as the amount of noise in the emission increases [59]. The noise-to-harmonic ratio measures the relative quantity of additional noise in the voice signal, which can be generated by the turbulence of the airflow in the glottis in cases of incomplete closure during phonation or also result from aperiodic vibration of the vocal folds [60], being associated with the presence of roughness. One of the limitations of this form of acoustic analysis is that, to perform a reliable analysis of jitter, shimmer, and noise measures, the sound signal cannot be too altered. This analysis is only reliable in normal or slightly altered voices, which prevents the evaluation of voices with more severe alterations.

3.3. Laryngeal features

Based on perceptual and acoustic data, many authors [3, 17, 33, 35, 61] state that individuals with hearing loss have difficulties in controlling the laryngeal function. To this date, however, laryngeal characteristics of individuals with hearing loss have not been thoroughly studied.

It has been stated that the larynx of a hearing-impaired child usually shows no anatomic or physiological abnormalities in the first years of life, but lack of auditory feedback can result in discoordination of intrinsic and extrinsic laryngeal muscles and disturbed contraction and relaxation of antagonistic muscles [13].

Inadequate laryngeal activity of four normally hearing and four hearing-impaired persons was found during productions of word-initial voiced and voiceless consonants with a flexible fiber-optic laryngoscope [62]. Three of the hearing-impaired subjects exhibited greater variability than their normally hearing peers in terms of the degree and duration of vocal fold abduction during voiceless consonant productions, but only one exhibited excessively wide glottal openings, suggesting that deaf persons waste air during speech production.

A study [63] was conducted with two normal hearing adults and four adults with profound hearing loss using high speed laryngeal film and acoustic data. The authors used the vowel-consonant-vowel segment "aha." The study found that two of the hearing-impaired subjects did not exhibit glottal waveforms in vowel production, which differed substantially from those of the normally hearing subjects. However, one subject with hearing loss exhibited maximal glottal openings approximately double those of the other subjects and large cycle-to-cycle variability. The most dramatic differences observed between the normally hearing and hearing-impaired subjects were the duration and the magnitude of the abductory gestures associated with devoicing. The vocal fold abductory-adductory movements associated with the devoiced segments appeared to be discontinuous in nature, which was characterized by abrupt abductory movement following the first vowel, which frequently reached a plateau before adductory movement associated with the second vowel. Such laryngeal features can result in abnormal voice production; however, these laryngeal findings were not correlated to voice quality.

3.4. Voice-related quality of life

The instruments used to measure quality of life in health sciences allow the understanding of the impact of a condition through patient perception. These materials have been used to obtain a multidimensional assessment of the human being. Patient-based assessment can be used to compose the evaluation process, helps clinicians to select strategies for rehabilitation based on specifics indentified, and monitors treatment outcomes [64].

With the inclusion of quality of life analysis in the health sciences, voice-related quality of life protocols were created since protocols about general health are not ideal to assess patients with voice disorders. Due to the importance of human communication in the several domains that contribute to quality of life, these instruments investigate if there are physical, emotional, and social limitations related to voice disorders, including the use of professional voice [65].

These instruments, therefore, contribute to the knowledge of the impact of the communication disorders manifested by the voice alteration. The extensive list of voice problems the individuals with hearing loss can affect their quality of life. However, the protocols of voice-related quality of life already developed are not entirely adequate to the voice problems frequently presented by individuals with hearing loss, and voice-related quality of life in individuals with hearing loss has not yet been thoroughly studied.

A single study [4] investigated voice-related quality of life in this population by comparing the scores of the Voice Handicap Index [66] between adults with moderate to profound hearing loss and their normal peers. There were significant differences in the total score and in the score of all three domains: functional, physical, and emotional. However, there was a major variability of responses obtained in the group of patients with hearing loss (a variation of 94 points) so the authors were not able to define a VHI score range.

Also, the several protocols of quality of life related to the presence of hearing loss or use of hearing aids [67–69] approach communication aspects regarding sound reception and not regarding the difficulties of voice and speech production, even though it is common knowledge that hearing interferes also in the emission stage of the communicative process.

4. Voice training in individuals with hearing loss

The auditory rehabilitation aims to allow deaf individuals using devices such as heading aids and cochlear implants to develop auditory abilities and oral communication. However, since voice characteristics commonly found in individuals with hearing loss can greatly compromise oral communication, voice training in addition to hearing, language, and speech rehabilitation is essential to restore normal physiology. For both prelingually deafened children and postlingually deafened adults, intervention can improve voice quality and prevent the development of abnormal voice production. Depending on the findings of the voice assessment, the treatment can include techniques for respiration, posture, movement of the articulators, vertical laryngeal excursion, loudness, and resonance [70].

The speech and language rehabilitation program of the Brasilia Teaching Hospital (Hospital Universitário de Brasília [HUB]) provides treatment for children, adolescents, and adults with moderate to profound hearing loss who are users of hearing aids and/or cochlear implants. The purpose of the therapy goes beyond speech perception. In the therapeutic plan, voice training is considered an element just as important as auditory training, being considered therefore a part of the extensive process of rehabilitation of individuals with hearing loss.

Voice training comprises many approaches: the universal methods that change voice quality as a whole and the specific techniques that rely on laryngeal imaging and aim to work with specific groups of muscles. With the use of different techniques and exercises, it is possible to modify the voice by acting on the muscle activity of the vocal tract, to enhance the relationship of the three subsystems of voice production (respiration, phonation, and resonance), and to demonstrate to the patient the many possibilities of motor adjustments of voice production

[57]. Based on the findings of the voice assessment and on laryngeal imaging whenever possible, the clinician can select a number of voice exercises that are thoroughly described in the literature [50, 71] to improve the abnormalities found. Some of the exercises suggested for hearing-impaired individuals are the prolonged /b/ exercise, manual circumlaryngeal massage associated with the emission of vowels and words, emissions of the closed vowels /o/ and /u/ while flexing the head to fix the larynx in a lower position, chewing, and lip vibration [72, 73]. In Table 3, some exercises for voice treatment [50, 71] are suggested based on findings of voice characteristics of individuals with hearing loss reported in the literature.

Voice feature	Purpose	Exercise
High fundamental frequency (f_0)	Reduce f_0, lower the larynx	Manual circumlaryngeal massage, yawn-sigh exercise, descendent pitch glide
High amplitude and frequency variation	Reduce amplitude and frequency variation	Visual monitoring of speech with computerized software
Nasality/resonance alterations	Increase intraoral air pressure, dissipate energy in the voice tract	Visual monitoring of nasal airflow with mirror or scape-scope, chewing exercises associated with vibratory sensations in nasal and facial bones, humming, mouth opening
Roughness, breathiness, harshness, strain	Balance aerodynamic and myoelastic forces, mobilize vocal fold mucosa	Manual circumlaryngeal massage, humming, chewing exercises, yawn-sigh exercise, tongue vibration, vocal fry
Instability	Improve phonatory stability	Exercises with long sustained tones
Monotone	Vary rate, pitch, and loudness	Musical scales, pitch glides, *messa di voce*, cards with arrows going up and down in a sentence
Excessive intonation	Promote control over pitch and loudness, reduce excessive vertical excursion of the larynx	Visual monitoring of speech using frequency and amplitude displays
Altered speech rate	Control speech rate	Monitor speech rate with metronome

Table 3. Common voice alterations in individuals with hearing loss and the respective techniques and exercises suggested in the voice rehabilitation.

Naturally, adapting the conventional voice therapy is very helpful, especially for people with severe to profound hearing loss since the training should not rely exclusively in auditory monitoring. Among the methods used for hearing rehabilitation is the multisensory method that uses the auditory channel, the visual channel, and tactile/kinesthetic cues [74, 75]. In the voice clinic, the use of visual, kinesthetic, and proprioceptive cues is extremely useful to develop parameters such as frequency and intensity [71], which is due to the fact that visual and tactile/kinetic feedbacks of the vocal apparatus are preserved in this population and should be explored in addition to the auditory training [70]. Abilities such as lip reading exemplify the use of visual cues for the development of speech and voice [72].

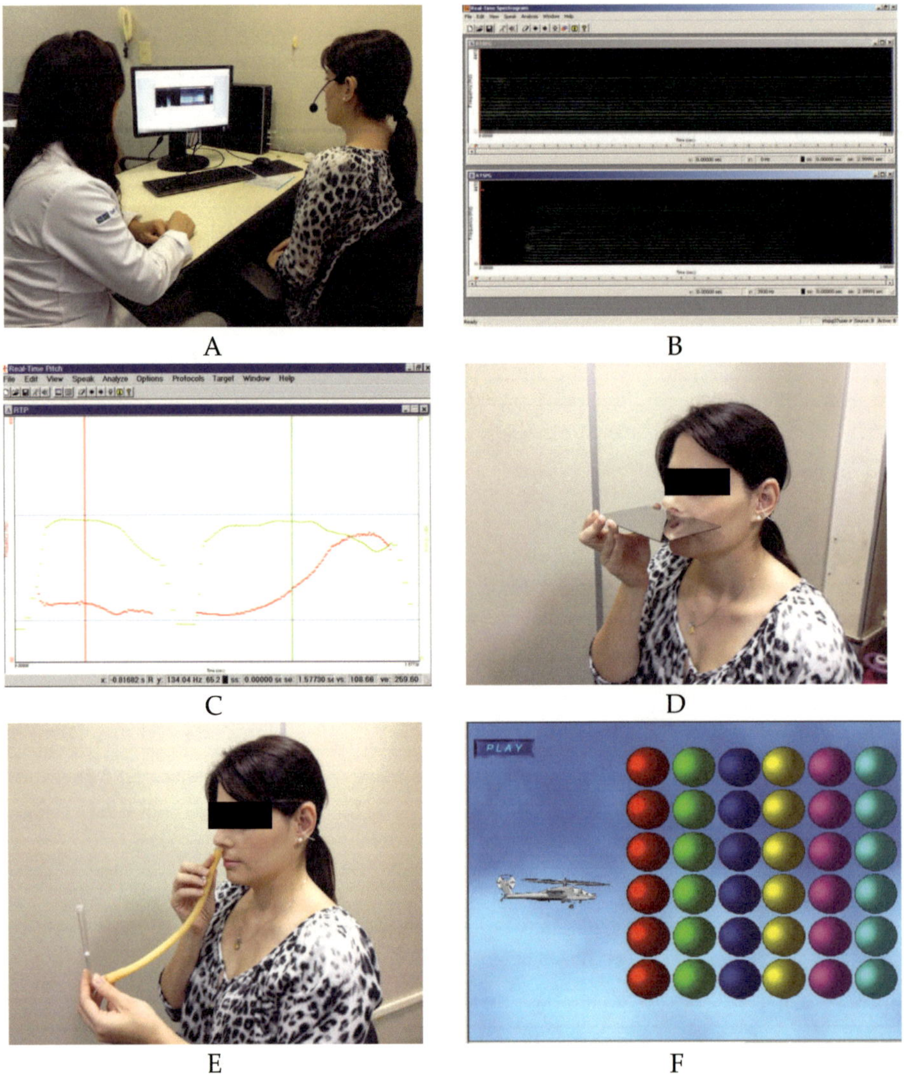

Figure 6. Examples of visual feedback in voice training. (A) Real-time spectrogram (GRAM 5.1.6). (B) Real-time monitoring of voice signal following a model provided in the upper window (Real Time Pitch, KayPentax). (C) Real-time monitoring of frequency and intensity. (D) Nasal mirror and for monitoring nasal airflow. (E) Scape-scope for monitoring nasal airflow. (F) Visual monitoring of intensity (Voice Games, KayPentax).

Using visual cues, it is possible to monitor adequate frequency and intensity with established thresholds, noise, voice attacks, strain, instability, formants, and voicing. Such methods are

http://dx.doi.org/10.5772/61217

considered effective in the voice rehabilitation of deaf individuals [76, 77]. Studies found improved frequency control, respiratory support, intelligibility, jitter and shimmer after voice therapy with computerized visual feedback [72, 78], and reduced nasality using visual cues to monitor nasal airflow [79, 80]. These cues include spectrograms, diagrams, nasal mirror, scape-scope, and even computerized software for children to promote a playful environment while training voice production (Figures 6A–6F).

The tactile/kinesthetic monitoring is harder to develop. Patients must identify proprioceptive symptoms and sensations that indicate abnormal voice production such as tightness, presence of secretion, pain, dryness, discomfort, etc. The procedure for using these cues include emission while touching the head, forehead, face, and resonance cavities, including the nose, neck, and thorax [71] (Figures 7A–7B).

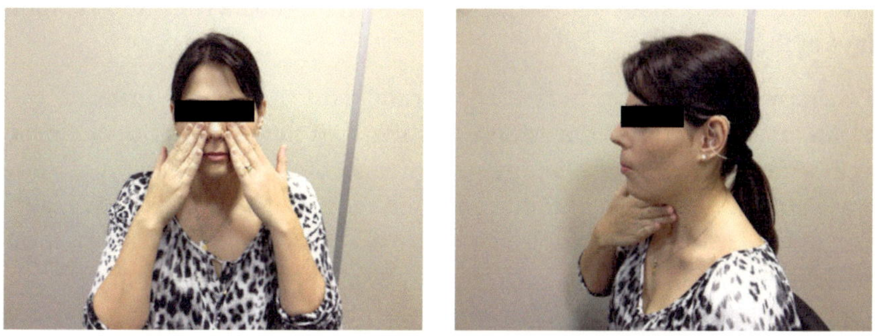

A B

Figure 7. Examples of kinesthetic feedback in voice training. (A) Hands feeling resonators for resonance control. (B) Monitoring larynx decent for normalizing pitch.

A structured voice therapy program for individual with hearing loss was described [78] and consisted of 16 therapy sessions, conducted twice a week with the duration of 1h. In the first half of the therapy session, the participants performed specific vocal exercises, which consisted of tongue snapping, tongue or lip vibration, humming, fricative sounds, prolonged /b/ exercise, vocal fry, overarticulation, chewing exercise, chanting, and visual/proprioceptive monitoring. In the second half, computerized games were used to provide visual feedback for monitoring frequency and intensity during speech tasks. The program showed promising results in speech and voice using these techniques and exercises. A similar approach was later suggested [72] using mainly visual feedback with computerized games and also finding improvement in speech and voice production.

A case study is presented to illustrate the immediate results of voice training during a therapy session of a young adult with profound hearing loss that use a unilateral cochlear implant. The patient is a 26-year-old male, with bilateral profound hearing loss due to bacterial meningitis at the age of 23 years.

To compare the results of the voice exercises, the prolonged /a/ vowel and a sample of sequential speech (counting from 1 to 10) were recorded pre- and post-therapy session. The perceptive analysis of the /a/ vowel pre-therapy evidenced brusque vocal attack, roughness, nasality, and instability. The sequential speech evidenced roughness, nasality, and imprecise articulation. The purpose of the voice exercises was to reduce laryngeal strain, to reduce nasality and cul-de-sac resonance improving relationship between glottal source and resonance, and to enhance articulation.

The selected exercises were as follows:

- Humming
- Humming associated with vowels
- Chanting the sequence "mananha, menenhe, mininhi, mononho, mununhu"
- Chewing exercise
- Chewing exercise associated with sequential speech (numbers from 1 to 10, months of the year, days of the week)

After the therapy session, there was a significant reduction of the brusque voice attack, roughness, and nasality in both emissions. In Table 4, some acoustics parameters of the /a/ vowel are presented pre- and post-therapy session using the Multi Dimensional Voice Program (MDVP, KayPentax). There was a slight reduction in fundamental frequency, although it is within normal standards for men at this age. There was also reduction of short- term variation (jitter) and long-term variation of frequency (jitter), short-term (shimmer) and long-term variation of amplitude (vAm), and reduction of the noise to harmonic ratio (NHR).

Parameter	Pre-therapy	Post-therapy
Average fundamental frequency (f_0)	127.052	123.322
Jitter (%)	3.966	3.337
Fundamental frequency variation (vF_0)	3.652	3.247
Shimmer (%)	5.590	4.176
Peak to peak amplitude variation (vAm)	14.535	9.725
Noise to harmonic ratio (NHR)	0.214	0.147

Table 4. Acoustic parameters of the /a/ vowel pre- and post-therapy session.

In Figure 8, the narrowband spectrogram of the pre-therapy /a/ vowel shows brusque voice attack, presence of subharmonics, low high-frequency harmonics, and instability. In the post-therapy spectrogram, increase in high-frequency harmonics, reduction of brusque voice attack, reduction of subharmonics, and reduction of instability are observed.

Figure 9 shows the narrowband spectrogram of the sequential speech using the Multi Speech Main Program (KayPentax), on which a significant increase of harmonics can be observed, although there is presence of subharmonics in both emissions.

http://dx.doi.org/10.5772/61217

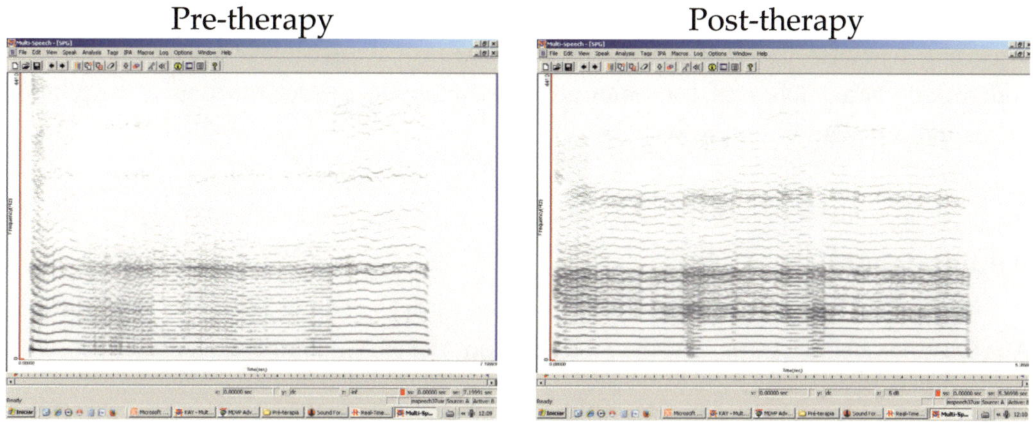

Figure 8. Spectrogram of the /a/ vowel pre- and post-therapy session.

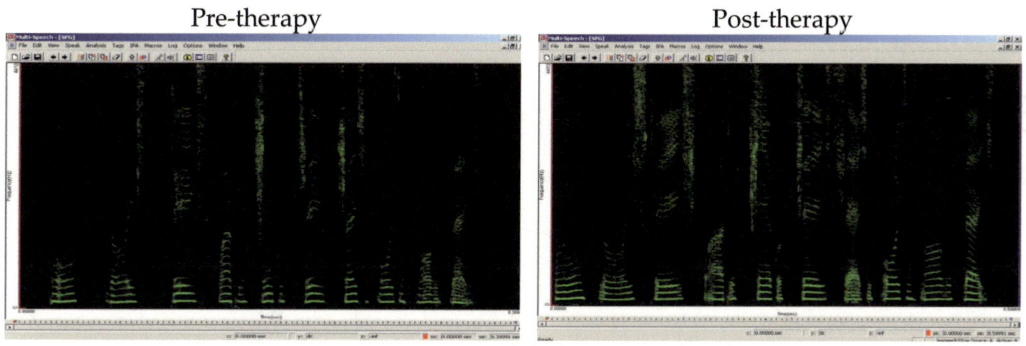

Figure 9. Spectrogram of the sequential speech pre- and post-therapy session.

This particulate case study showed that voice training was helpful to improve voice production and consequently oral communication. The acoustic and perceptual characteristics of this individual improved significantly, and the most prominent features were improvement of resonance and instability.

5. Conclusions

The primary difficulties of children and adults with hearing loss are related to auditory abilities and language development, and with reason, they become the primary center of attention in the rehabilitation process. However, voice abnormalities should not be overlooked since they can greatly compromise voice quality and speech intelligibility. There is still much to be done in this area of expertise. The understanding of laryngeal behavior, acoustic and perceptual characteristics, voice-related quality of life, and an effective implementation of voice training in the process of rehabilitation is crucial. In adequate proportions, vocal rehabilitation should take place along with the auditory training and oral language development since the very beginning of treatment so that individuals with hearing loss can achieve intelligible, pleasant, and socially acceptable oral communication, maintaining correct function of respiration, phonation, articulation, and resonance.

Author details

Ana Cristina Coelho[1*], Daniela Malta Medved[1] and Alcione Ghedini Brasolotto[2]

*Address all correspondence to: anacrisccoelho@yahoo.com.br

1 Brasília Teaching Hospital, University of Brasília, Brasília-DF, Brazil

2 Department of Speech-Language and Audiology, Bauru School of Dentistry, University of São Paulo, Bauru-SP, Brazil

References

[1] Ubrig MT, Goffi-Gomez MV, Weber R, Menezes MH, Nemr NK, Tsuji DH, et al. Voice analysis of postlingually deaf adults pre- and postcochlear implantation. J Voice. 2011;25(6):692–9.

[2] Hassan SM, Malki KH, Mesallam TA, Farahat M, Bukhari M, Murry T. The effect of cochlear implantation on nasalance of speech in postlingually hearing–impaired adults. J Voice. 2012;26(5):669.e17–22.

[3] Behlau M, Thomé R, Azevedo R, Rehder MI, Thomé DC. Disfonias congênitas. In: Behlau M. Voz: O livro do especialista. Rio de Janeiro: Revinter; 2005. pp. 1–50.

[4] Voz: fonoaudiologia e medicina. FOB–USP/UNIFESP/FM–USP. 2006. [CD–ROM] São Paulo: FOB–USP/UNIFESP/FM–USP; 2006.

[5] American Speech-Language-Hearing Association. ASHA: Understanding voice production. http://voicefoundation.org/health–science/voice–disorders/anatomy–physiology–of–voice–production/understanding–voice–production/ (accessed 24 June 2015).

[6] Argentim JP. Cross–cultural translation and adaptation of the Virtual Man Project's CD–ROM "Voice assessment: speech–language pathology and audiology & medicine, " Vol.1 to American English Language. Master's dissertation. University of São Paulo; 2013.

[7] Madeira FB, Tomita S. Voice Handicap Index evaluation in patients with moderate to profound bilateral sensorineural hearing loss. Braz J Otorhinolaryngol. 2010;76(1):59–70.

[8] Buder EH, Chorna LB, Oller DK, Robinson RB. Vibratory regime classification of infant phonation. J Voice. 2008;22(5):553–64.

[9] Baraldi GoS, Castro de Almeida L, Calais LL, Borges AC, Gielow I, Raymundo De Cunto M. Study of the fundamental frequency in elderly women with hearing loss. Braz J Otorhinolaryngol. 2007;73(3):378–83.

[10] Selleck MA, Sataloff RT. The impact of the auditory system on phonation: a review. J Voice. 2014;28(6):688–93.

[11] Tourville JA, Reilly KJ, Guenther FH. Neural mechanisms underlying auditory feedback control of speech. Neuroimage. 2008;39(3):1429–43.

[12] Jones JA, Keough D. Auditory-motor mapping for pitch control in singers and nonsingers. Exp Brain Res. 2008;190(3):279–87.

[13] Das B, Chatterjee I, Kumar S. Laryngeal aerodynamics in children with hearing impairment versus age and height matched normal hearing peers. ISRN Otolaryngol. 2013;2013:394–604.

[14] Baudonck N, Van Lierde K, D'haeseleer E, Dhooge I. A comparison of the perceptual evaluation of speech production between bilaterally implanted children, unilaterally implanted children, children using hearing aids, and normal-hearing children. Int J Audiol. 2011;50(12):912–9.

[15] Van Lierde KM, Vinck BM, Baudonck N, De Vel E, Dhooge I. Comparison of the overall intelligibility, articulation, resonance, and voice characteristics between children using cochlear implants and those using bilateral hearing aids: a pilot study. Int J Audiol. 2005;44(8):452–65.

[16] Baudonck N, Van Lierde K, Dhooge I, Corthals P. A comparison of vowel productions in prelingually deaf children using cochlear implants, severe hearing-impaired children using conventional hearing aids and normal-hearing children. Folia Phoniatr Logop. 2011;63(3):154–60.

[17] Baudonck N, D'haeseleer E, Dhooge I, Van Lierde K. Objective vocal quality in children using cochlear implants: a multiparameter approach. J Voice. 2011;25(6):683–91.

[18] Higgins MB, Carney AE, Schulte L. Physiological assessment of speech and voice production of adults with hearing loss. J Speech Hear Res. 1994;37(3):510–21.

[19] Campisi P, Low A, Papsin B, Mount R, Cohen-Kerem R, Harrison R. Acoustic analysis of the voice in pediatric cochlear implant recipients: a longitudinal study. Laryngoscope. 2005;115(6):1046–50.

[20] Hocevar-Boltezar I, Radsel Z, Vatovec J, Geczy B, Cernelc S, Gros A, et al. Change of phonation control after cochlear implantation. Otol Neurotol. 2006;27(4):499–503.

[21] Evans MK, Deliyski DD. Acoustic voice analysis of prelingually deaf adults before and after cochlear implantation. J Voice. 2007;21(6):669–82.

[22] Campisi P, Low AJ, Papsin BC, Mount RJ, Harrison RV. Multidimensional voice program analysis in profoundly deaf children: quantifying frequency and amplitude control. Percept Mot Skills. 2006;103(1):40–50.

[23] Holler T, Campisi P, Allegro J, Chadha NK, Harrison RV, Papsin B, et al. Abnormal voicing in children using cochlear implants. Arch Otolaryngol Head Neck Surg. 2010;136(1):17–21.

[24] Souza LB, Bevilacqua MC, Brasolotto AG, Coelho AC. Cochlear implanted children present vocal parameters within normal standards. Int J Pediatr Otorhinolaryngol. 2012;76(8):1180–3.

[25] Lee GC, Liu C, Lee SH. Effects of hearing aid amplification on voice F0 variability in speakers with prelingual hearing loss. Hear Res. 2013;302:1–8.

[26] Coelho AC, Brasolotto AG, Bevilacqua MC. An initial study of voice characteristics of children using two different sound coding strategies in comparison to normal hearing children. Int J Audiol. 2015:1–7.

[27] Nguyen LH, Allegro J, Low A, Papsin B, Campisi P. Effect of cochlear implantation on nasality in children. Ear Nose Throat J. 2008;87(3):138, 40–3.

[28] Wirz S. The voice of the deaf. In: Fawcus M. Voice Disorders and Their Management. 2nd edition. San Diego: Singular; 1991. pp. 283–303.

[29] Perrin E, Berger–Vachon C, Topouzkhanian A, Truy E, Morgon A. Evaluation of cochlear implanted children's voices. Int J Pediatr Otorhinolaryngol. 1999;47(2):181–6.

[30] Baudonck N, Van Lierde K, D'haeseller, Dhooge, I. Nasalance and nasality in children with cochlear implants and children with hearing aids. Int J Pediatr Otorhinolaryngol [Journal on the interner]. 2015 Jan 29 [cited 2015 mar 6]. doi: 10.1016/j.ijporl.2015.01.025. [Epub ahead of print].

[31] Mora R, Crippa B, Cervoni E, Santomauro V, Guastini L. Acoustic features of voice in patients with severe hearing loss. J Otolaryngol Head Neck Surg. 2012;41(1):8–13.

[32] Valero Garcia J, Rovira JM, Sanvicens LG. The influence of the auditory prosthesis type on deaf children's voice quality. Int J Pediatr Otorhinolaryngol. 2010;74(8):843–8.

[33] Hocevar-Boltezar I, Vatovec J, Gros A, Zargi M. The influence of cochlear implantation on some voice parameters. Int J Pediatr Otorhinolaryngol. 2005;69(12):1635–40.

[34] Seifert E, Oswald M, Bruns U, Vischer M, Kompis M, Haeusler R. Changes of voice and articulation in children with cochlear implants. Int J Pediatr Otorhinolaryngol. 2002;66(2):115–23.

[35] Guerrero Lopez HA, Mondain M, Amy de la Bretèque B, Serrafero P, Trottier C, Barkat-Defradas M. Acoustic, aerodynamic, and perceptual analyses of the voice of cochlear-implanted children. J Voice. 2013;27(4):523.e1–17.

[36] Allegro J, Papsin BC, Harrison RV, Campisi P. Acoustic analysis of voice in cochlear implant recipients with post-meningitic hearing loss. Cochlear Implants Int. 2010;11(2):100–16.

[37] Van Lierde KM, Vinck BM, Baudonck N, De Vel E, Dhooge I. Comparison of the overall intelligibility, articulation, resonance, and voice characteristics between children using cochlear implants and those using bilateral hearing aids: a pilot study. Int J Audiol. 2005;44(8):452–65.

[38] Horga D, Liker M. Voice and pronunciation of cochlear implant speakers. Clin Linguist Phon. 2006;20(2–3):211–7.

[39] Eskander A, Gordon KA, Tirado Y, Hopyan T, Russell L, Allegro J, et al. Normal-like motor speech parameters measured in children with long-term cochlear implant experience using a novel objective analytic technique. JAMA Otolaryngol Head Neck Surg. 2014;140(10):967–74.

[40] Lee GS. Variability in voice fundamental frequency of sustained vowels in speakers with sensorineural hearing loss. J Voice. 2012;26(1):24–9.

[41] Lejska M. Voice field measurements-a new method of examination: the influence of hearing on the human voice. J Voice. 2004;18(2):209–15.

[42] Laver J. The Phonetic Description of Voice Quality. London: Cambridge University Press; 1980. pp. 184–208.

[43] Hirano M. Clinical Examination of Voice. New York: Springer–Verlag; 1981. pp. 81–4.

[44] Dejonckere P, Remacle M, Freznel-Elbaz E. Reliability and relevance of differentiated perceptual evaluation of pathological voice quality. In: Clemente MP. Voice Update. Amsterdam: Elsevier; 1996. pp. 321–4.

[45] Shriberg LD, Kwiatkowski J, Rasmusen C. The Prosody-Voice Screening Profile (PVSP). Tucson: AZ Communication Skill Builder; 1990.

[46] ASHA. Consensus Auditory-Perceptual Evaluation of Voice (CAPE-V) Special Interest Division 3, Voice and Voice Disorders. http://www.asha.org (accessed February 1, 2015).

[47] Simberg S, Laine A, Sala E, Rönnemaa AM. Prevalence of voice disorders among future teachers. J Voice. 2000;14:231–35.

[48] Lenden JM, Flipsen Jr P, Prosody and voice characteristics of children with cochlear implants. J Commun Disord. 2007;40(1):66–81.

[49] Ysunza A, Vazquez MC. Velopharyngeal sphincter physiology in deaf individuals. Cleft Palate Craniofac J. 1993;30(2):141–3.

[50] Boone D, McFarlane S. The Voice and Voice Therapy. Englewood-Cliff: Prentice Hall; 1988.

[51] Subtelny JD, Whitehead RL, Samar VJ. Spectral study of deviant resonance in the speech of women who are deaf. J Speech Hear Res. 1992;35(3):574–9.

[52] Fletcher SG, Mahfuz F, Hendarmin HH. Nasalance in the speech of children with normal hearing and children with hearing loss. Am J Speech Lang Pathol. 1999;8:241–8.

[53] Nakata T, Trehub SE, Kanda Y. Effect of cochlear implants on children's perception and production of speech prosody. J Acoust Soc Am. 2012;131(2):1307–14.

[54] Peng SC, Tomblin JB, Turner CW. Production and perception of speech intonation in pediatric cochlear implant recipients and individuals with normal hearing. Ear Hear. 2008;29(3):336–51.

[55] Chin SB, Bergeson TR, Phan J. Speech intelligibility and prosody production in children with cochlear implants. J Commun Disord. 2012;45(5):355–66.

[56] Giusti MC, Padovani MMP, Behlau M, Granato L. The voice of hearing impaired children. Braz J Otorhinolaringol. 2001;67:29–35.

[57] Baken RJ, Orlikoff RF. Speech movements. In: Baken RJ, Orlikoff RF. Clinical Measurement Speech and Voice. 2nd ed. San Diego: Singular Thomson Learning; 2000. pp. 511–57.

[58] Dehqan A, Scherer RC. Objective voice analysis of boys with profound hearing loss. J Voice. 2011;25(2):e61–5.

[59] Behlau M, Madazio G, Feijo D, Pontes P. Avaliação de Voz. In: Behlau, M. Voz: o Livro do Especialista. Rio de Janeiro: Revinter. 2001. pp.105–15.

[60] Ferrand, C. Harmonics-to-noise ratio: an index of vocal aging. J Voice. 2002;16(4): 480–7.

[61] Wirz SL, Subtelny JD, Whitehead RL. Perceptual and spectrographic study of tense voice in normal hearing and deaf subjects. Folia Phoniatr (Basel). 1981;33(1):23–36.

[62] Mahshie JJ, Conture EG. Deaf speakers' laryngeal behavior. J Speech Hear Res. 1983;26(4):550–9.

[63] Metz DE, Whitehead RL, Whitehead BH. Mechanics of vocal fold vibration and laryngeal articulatory gestures produced by hearing–impaired speakers. J Speech Hear Res. 1984;27(1):62–9.

[64] Behlau M, Alves Dos Santos LeM, Oliveira G. Cross-cultural adaptation and validation of the voice handicap index into Brazilian Portuguese. J Voice. 2011;25(3):354–9.

[65] Madazio G, Moreti F, Yamasaki R. Protocolos de Autoavaliação do Impacto da Disfonia. In: Marquesan IQ, Silva HJ, Tomé MC. (3rd ed.) Tratado das Especialidades em Fonoaudiologia. São Paulo: Roca; 2014. pp. 113–26.

[66] Jacobson BH, Johnson A, Grywalski C, Silbergleit A, Jacobson G, Benninger M, et al. The voice handicap index (VHI): development and validation. Amer J Speech Lang Pathol. 1997; 6:66–70.

[67] Fleck MPA, Louzada S, Xavier M, Chachamovich, E, Vieria G, Santos V, et al. Application of the Portuguese version of the abbreviated instrument of quality life WHOQOL–bref. Rev Saúde Pública. 2000;34(2):178–83.

[68] Rosis ACA, Souza MRF, Iório MCM. Questionnaire Hearing Handicap Inventory for the Elderly–Screening version (HHIE–S): sensitivity and specificity study. Rev Soc Bras Fonoaudiol. 2009;14(3):339–45.

[69] Newman CW1, Weinstein BE, Jacobson GP, Hug GA.The Hearing Handicap Inventory for Adults: psychometric adequacy and audiometric correlates. Ear Hear. 1990 Dec;11(6):430–3.

[70] Pinho, S. Proposal of voice evaluation in hearing impaired. Pró-fono. 1990;2(1):17–9.

[71] Behlau M, Madazio G, Feijó D, Azevedo R, Gielow I, Rehder MI. Aperfeiçoamento vocal e tratamento fonoaudiológico das disfonias. In: Behlau M. Voz: O livro do especialista. Rio de Janeiro: Revinter; 2005. pp. 409–525.

[72] Lopes DCJ. Evaluation of voice and speech intelligibility of deaf individuals before and after speech therapy utilizing computerized resources. Master's dissertation. São Paulo: University of São Paulo; 2004.

[73] Souza LB, Bevilacqua MC. A efetividade de técnicas vocais na terapia de voz do usuário de Implante Coclear. Proceedings of the 19 o Congresso Brasileiro e 8o internacional de fonoaudiologia; 2011 Oct 30–Sep 1; São Paulo, SP. São Paulo: SBFa; 2011.

[74] Cárnio MS, Couto MIV, Lichtig I. Linguagem e surdez. In: Lacerda CBF, Nakamura H, Lima MC, organizadoras. Fonoaudiologia: surdez e abordagem bilíngue. São Paulo: Plexus; 2000. pp. 44–55.

[75] Sarwat A, Baraka S, Bassiouny M, Saleh E, Saber A. Kinesthetic versus auditory cues in speech monitoring of post-lingual cochlear implant patients. International Congress Series 1240. 2003; pp. 417–21.

[76] Oliveira PMT. Auxílio visual à oralização dos surdos [Master's dissertation]. Rio de Janeiro: Federal University of Rio de Janeiro; 1998.

[77] Araújo AML. Jogos Computacionais Fonoarticulatórios para Crianças com Deficiência Auditiva. PhD thesis. Campinas: University of Campinas; 2000.

[78] Bommarito S. The effect of a voice therapy method on vocal quality and speech intelligibility in deaf individuals. PhD thesis. São Paulo: Federal University of São Paulo; 2000.

[79] Junqueira P, Vaz ACN, Peyres LC, Pignatari SN, Weckx LLM. Management of hypernasality caused by adenoidectomy. Rev Bras Otorrinolaringol. 2002;68(4):593–6.

[80] Melo DP, Ramalho MSSC, Perillo VCA, Rodrigues LCB. Intensive speech therapy and cleft palate: case report. Rev CEFAC. 2013;15(4):1019–24.

Section 3

Noise Induced Hearing Loss

Chapter 7

Hearing Impairment in Professional Musicians and Industrial Workers — Profession-Specific Auditory Stimuli Used to Evoke Event-Related Brain Potentials and to Show Different Auditory Perception and Processing

Edeltraut Emmerich, Marcus Engelmann, Melanie Rohmann and Frank Richter

Additional information is available at the end of the chapter

http://dx.doi.org/10.5772/61137

Abstract

Hearing impaired professional musicians or industrial workers often report that they were able to identify mistuned chords in a music piece or even slight changes in the noise of their machines (usually > 100 dB SPL) though they were handicapped in listening tasks in daily routine.

In order to assess central processing of acoustic stimuli, we analyzed auditory evoked potentials (AEP) and EEG spectra after stimulation with work-related auditory stimuli in healthy controls, in hearing impaired musicians or hearing impaired workers from the beverage industry. Stimuli were series of in-tune or mistuned synthetic piano chords or the original machine noise the workers heard in daily routine and the same noise with disturbing signals.

Professional musicians identified the mistuned stimuli and the AEP differed significantly. The workers recognized the disturb signals. In both groups the spectral analysis confirmed a frequency shift towards higher alpha frequencies and an altered spatial distribution of the EEG frequencies during presentation of the disturb signals.

We assume that professionalism causes learning of typical auditory stimuli that is important for auditory processing after hearing impairment. AEP component analysis and spectral analysis of the EEG are important tools to objectify this processing, in particular in hearing impaired employees.

Keywords: Auditory evoked potential, Mismatch negativity (MMN), Hearing impairment, Permanent threshold shift (PTS), Occupational disease

1. Introduction

The mismatch negativity component (MMN) of auditory evoked event-related potential can be elicited by deviant stimuli inserted into a follow-up of identical sounds [1]. See for review [2]. In the past, numerous studies had been performed in which changed attributes of the stimuli, such as decrement in duration [3], changes in frequency [4], or changed stimulus intensity [5], were used to differentiate between standard and deviant stimuli. MMN to musical stimuli has been investigated for a long time. It was shown that MMN was caused by a timbre change [6,7]. In a later study, it was shown [8] that comparison of MMN to omitted tones in a series of sine-wave tone pips could be used to differentiate between musicians and non-musicians. Violation of harmony rules elicited large MMN in the fronto-central cortex areas [9]. Slightly mistuned chords produced MMN in professional violinists, but not in non-musicians [10]. Similarly, larger and earlier MMN to rhythm variations were observed in jazz musicians than in non-musicians [11].

An earlier study of our group raised the issue that hearing-impaired professional musicians were able to play their instruments in the orchestras and to perform without problems when they were trained for years, regardless of their permanent threshold shift (PTS) [12]. Interestingly, those musicians reported on hearing problems when watching TV or if they wanted to have conversation in a noisy environment (party-noise effect). To our knowledge, there are only few studies about musicians dealing with the effects of occupational noise and central compensation after hearing damage. Therefore, we want to test whether differences exist in auditory event-related potentials (AEP) (amplitudes and latencies) and/or in MMN reflecting the sound processing while comparing normal hearing people and musicians (normal hearing and hearing impaired). The new aspect in our study is the use of typical musical stimuli, i.e., in-tune and mistuned chords. We assumed that professional musicians should be trained to these stimuli regardless whether they have normal hearing or not.

There is some evidence for the assumption that ongoing training of professional musicians would produce changes in the central processing of musical auditory signals since an earlier study did not find different neural generators for MMN while comparing musicians and non-musicians, but found typical differences in MMN between both groups after omitted tone pips [8]. From other data, it was supposed that ongoing professional training could result in a more accurate tuning of frequency-specific neurons in musicians [10]. Professional musicians are considered to be a model for cortical plasticity caused by ongoing musical training [13-17]. In a review [18], it was summarized that top-down and bottom-up plasticity exists in the auditory cortex, as well as in other somatosensory areas of the brain. This was supported by a recent study [19] that showed that the posterior medial cortex is involved in processing of melodic and harmonic information. If ongoing musical training participates in this process, it would be interesting to see whether a hearing deficit in trained professional musicians would interfere with, e.g., an improved tuning function or with the recognition of wrongly tuned sounds.

The present experiments investigated whether MMN could be detected in professional musicians, non-musicians, or industrial workers without formal musical training when typical musical stimuli (C-chords) were presented in the oddball-design. To get better information over the whole range of audibility, we applied the stimuli both in the mid-frequency and in the high-frequency range. We analyzed the amplitudes and latencies of the first positive and negative components of the AEP. We looked further for differences in the MMN between the three investigated groups. In another series of experiments, we tested with the same paradigm, whether MMN to mistuned high-frequency stimuli could still be observed in hearing-impaired professional musicians with a PTS in the high-frequency range between 3.000 Hz and 8.000 Hz. To evaluate to what extent the subjects were annoyed by the mistuned chords, we analyzed the EEG frequency activity in the interstimulus intervals and additionally looked for changes in heart frequency. To check, whether a long-lasting professional training might have induced a learning process for specific sounds, we repeated the EEG and heart frequency analysis in the group of hearing-impaired workers and presented them slightly disturbed machine noise they usually had heard in their daily working routine.

Hypotheses:

1. Ongoing professional training of musicians or of workers to listen to specific sounds either while performing music or watching machine sounds changes the central sound processing. These changes in AEP can be used to differentiate between untrained and trained persons.

2. The ongoing training to profession-specific sounds enables the trained person to recognize even slight deviations. The recognition is reflected by specific late components of the AEP, even when the person was not aware of the deviated stimulus.

3. The learned specific sounds could even be recognized when sound perception is disturbed by a permanent hearing impairment (PTS). External stimuli that were not trained would not be recognized even though they would be presented in the same sound intensity.

2. Materials and methods

2.1. Proband groups

Normal hearing and hearing-impaired non-musicians, aged 16 to 30 years

A group consisting of 16 members of the Medical Faculty of Jena (mean age 21.3 years) who had no hearing deficits, and who did not perform music regularly and never had formal training in music was categorized as non-musicians. The participants were all right-handed.

The hearing-impaired group (10 age-matched participants) had a hearing deficit (PTS) of about 20 dB SPL in the frequency range from 3.000 Hz to 8.000 Hz.

Normal hearing and hearing-impaired professional musicians, aged 28 to 68 years

In this part of the study participated 15 professional normal hearing musicians (mean age 41.4 years) who were employed at three German orchestras. The instrument groups were violins, trombones, oboes, bassoons, cellos, violas, and contrabasses. A second group of 10 professional musicians from the same three orchestras (mean age 48.1 years) had a hearing deficit (PTS) of more than 30 dB in frequencies larger 3 kHz. These 10 musicians played violins, contrabasses, bassoon, cello, trombones, and oboe.

Hearing-impaired industrial workers, aged 38 to 63 years

In this part of the study participated 20 industrial workers from a brewery who worked on bottle washing or bottle filling machines. Their hearing loss (PTS) of more than 20 dB SPL in the frequency range from 3.000 Hz to 8.000 Hz was officially recognized as an occupational disease. The workers were aged 38 to 63 years and had never had formal musical training or played any kind of music. All experiments were performed without hearing aids.

2.2. Study design

The study was approved by the local ethics committee of the University of Jena. All participants gave informed consent to this study and received monetary compensation for their participation. In a questionnaire, the participants were asked for their age; musical experiences, i.e., duration of employment in the orchestra or attending music school, instruments that are or were played, duration of training time per week, and the use of hearing protectors; occurrence of tinnitus; occurrence of ear, nose, and throat diseases; and hereditary ear diseases in the family. We also asked for noisy leisure time activities. The workers were asked similar questions with special respect for noise exposition per working shift. The hearing ability of the right and left ears in each participant was tested by means of a high frequency audiometer (Grahnert Präcitronic MA 22; Dresden, Germany, combined with a headphone HDA-200; Sennheiser, Hannover, Germany) and by measuring the otoacoustic emissions (DPOAE/TEOAE) (Madsen, Denmark). Details were given by our group in the literature [12].

To study the perception of auditory stimuli, we recorded MMN using the classical ac-EEG technique. Participants were seated comfortably with closed eyes. They listened to the stimuli that were presented via loudspeakers in the free field mode and were instructed only to listen relaxed and to avoid attention or any reaction to the stimuli to minimize artifacts caused by movements.

The ac-EEG was recorded from 32 electrodes (Figure 1) positioned according to the international 10/20 system over frontal, central, temporal and parietal brain areas of both hemispheres using the standardized Easy-Cap device (Easy Cap GmbH, Herrsching-Breitbrunn, Germany). A linked-mastoid electrode served as a reference. Impedance was maintained below 5 kOhm. An electrode at the forehead was used as a ground. The electrooculogram was recorded for rejection of artifacts (two electrodes above and below the eye, one electrode lateral to the eye).

http://dx.doi.org/10.5772/61137

The EEG was recorded with the Brain Products recording system (Brain Products GmbH, Gilching, Germany). The bandpass ranged from 0.1 Hz to 250 Hz. The amplified signals were digitized at a 5.000 Hz sample rate and analyzed off-line. The electrocardiogram was recorded for a beat-to-beat frequency analysis.

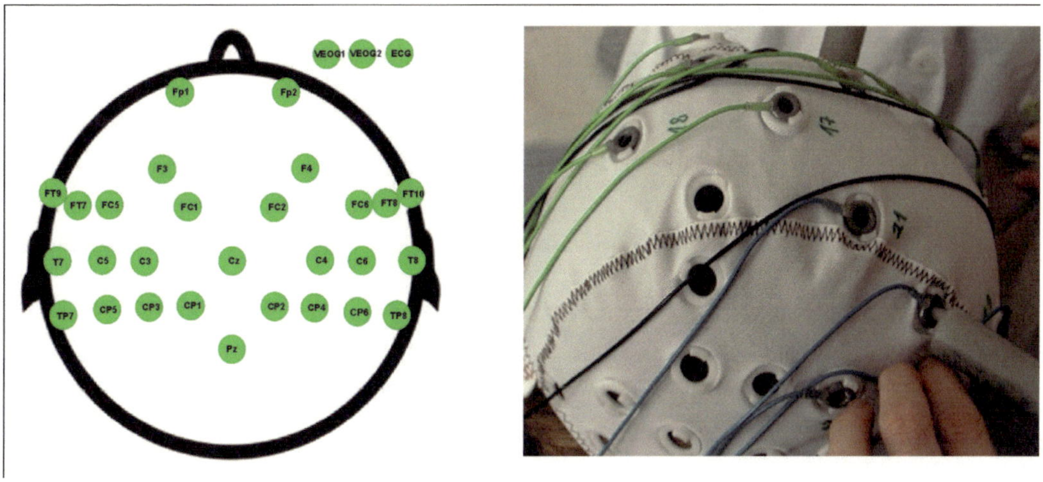

Figure 1. The left panel shows the typical electrode positions at the cap that were used in this study. Two additional reference electrodes were placed at the mastoids and as a ground electrode, the FPC position was used. To extract artifacts by eye movements, the VEOG was recorded with two electrodes. For analyzing the heart rate, the electrocardiogram in the Einthoven triangle was recorded (symbolized by the ECG marking). The right panel shows the Easy Cap device on the head while fixing the electrodes.

2.3. Auditory stimuli

Stimuli were pure C1-major chords, C3 chords, and respective mistuned chords in a classical oddball paradigm. The mistuned chords were generated by a synthesizer (variation +50 cent of the middle tone for the C-major chord, and variation +12 cent for the C3 chord) (Figure 2). A frequency and spectrogram analysis was performed to assure that the mistuned chords were in the same frequency range and had a similar intensity (integrating-averaging Sound Level Meter, type 118, class 1; Norsonic, Lierskog, Norway). Whereas the +50 cent variation was easy to differentiate from correct tunes, the +12 cent variation was difficult to discern for all non-trained listeners.

Stimuli were stored on a PC and presented in a free-field mode via the Presentation software (Presentation V9.12, NBS, Berkeley, CA) via two active loudspeakers as shown in Figure 3.

A recording session consisted of four trains per 200 single stimuli each. The participants listened with closed eyes to two trains of C1-major chords and to two trains of C3 chords. Parent and deviant stimuli were presented randomly in a 4:1 order and at randomized interstimulus intervals lasting from 2 to 6 seconds. We defined three different paradigms of stimulus occurrence: paradigm 1 had 150 normal and 50 mistuned C1-major chords, paradigm

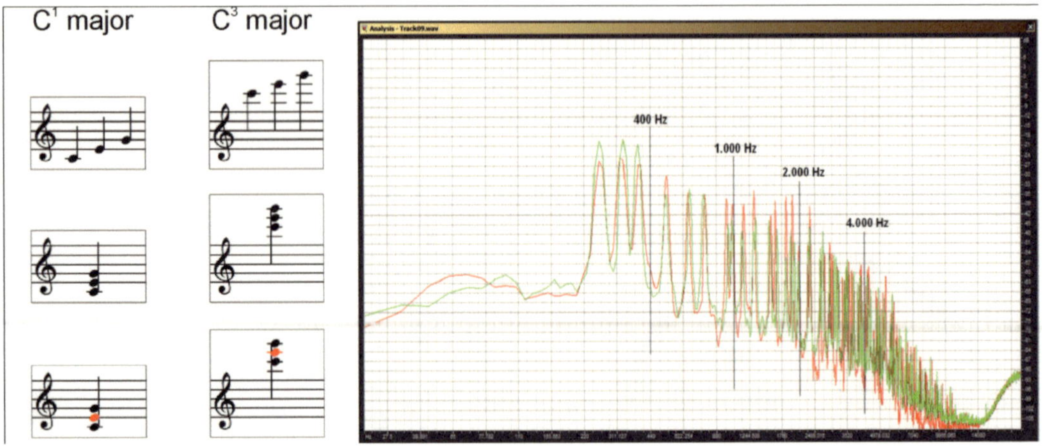

Figure 2. Design of the musical chords produced with a computer synthesizer. The C1 major (ca. 400 Hz) were the low frequency stimuli and the C3 major (ca. 1300 Hz) the high frequency stimuli. For mistuning, the middle tone E was modified (marked with red in the lower panels on the left side). The diagram on the right shows a screenshot with the intensities of both stimuli in a frequency spectrum. Note that there is no significant difference in intensity between the normal and mistuned stimuli.

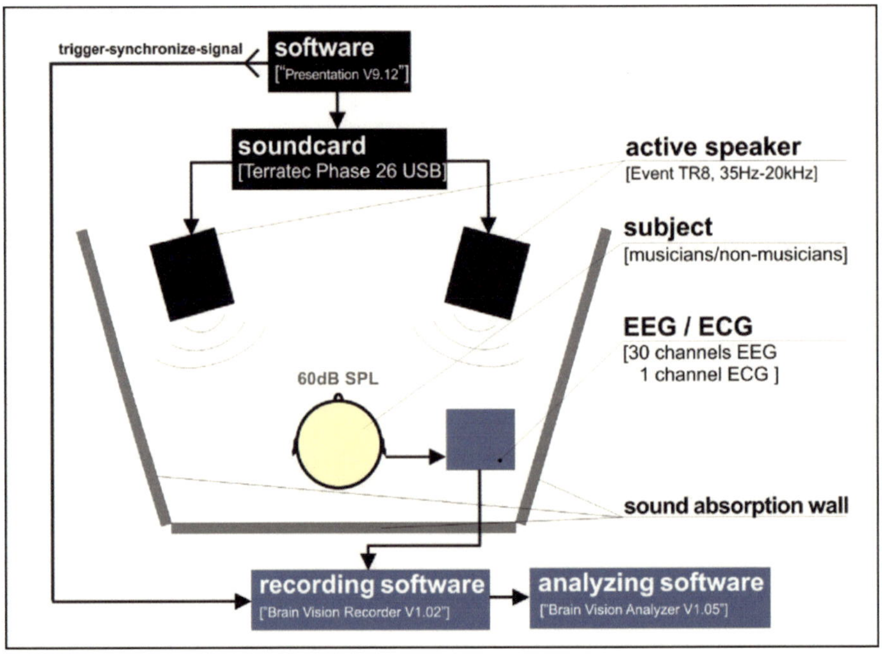

Figure 3. Schematic diagram of sound presentation and data recording setup in this study.

2 150 mistuned and 50 normal C1-major chords, and paradigm 3 150 normal and 50 mistuned C3-major chords. Non-musicians and professional musicians listened to all three paradigms. The stimulus intensity was set at 65 dB SPL.

The industrial workers listened only to musical stimuli in the paradigms 1 and 2 with the same number of stimuli. For testing the industrial workers with specific sounds they were trained to listen to we recorded samples of the machine noise as parent stimuli and interrupted this machine noise with short high-pitched whistles or with very short intervals of random white noise (deviant stimulus). Both types of stimuli were presented in an oddball paradigm with similar time intervals at an intensity of 65 dB SPL.

2.4. Data analysis

Trials contaminated with artifacts (e.g., contractions of mimic muscles or eye movements) were excluded from further analysis. The AEP in the EEG were evaluated using the BrainVision Analyzer 2 (Brain Products, Munich, Germany). We observed a 512 ms time range with a 50 ms pre-stimulus interval. A set of raw EEG data from all electrodes is presented in Figure 4.

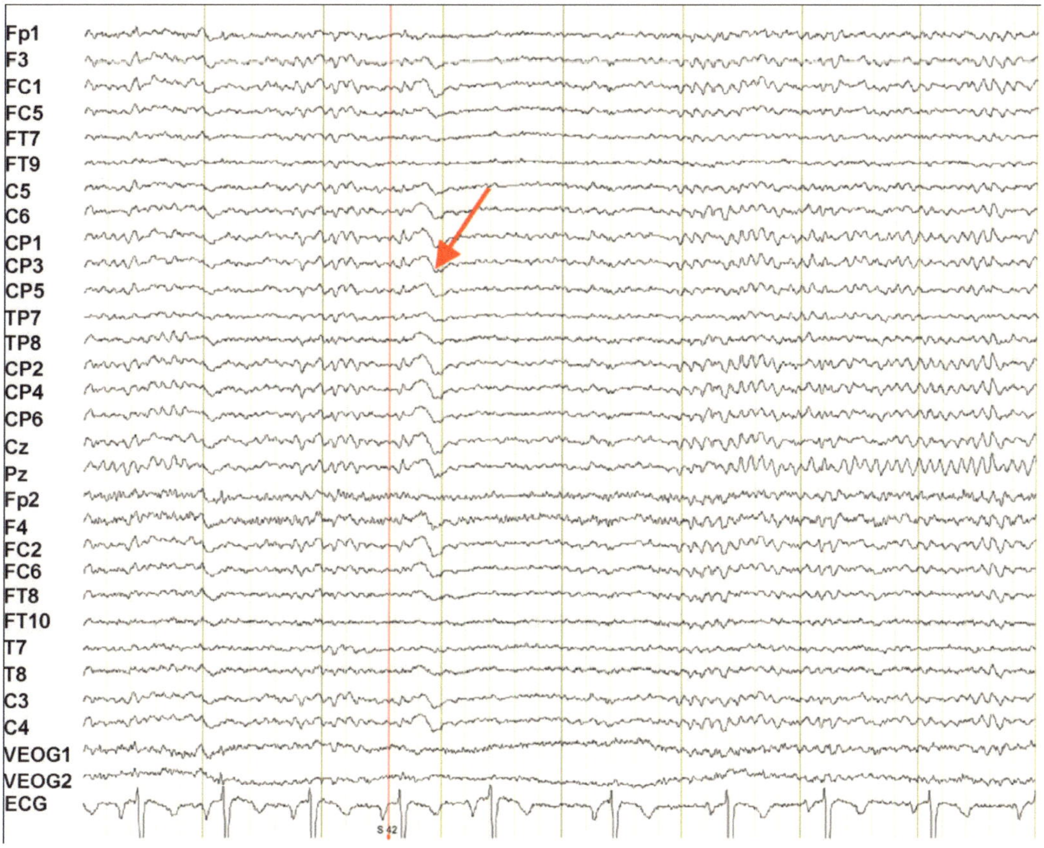

Figure 4. Specimen of an EEG recording, the recordings of EOG and of electrocardiogram with presentation of an auditory stimulus marked by the red dot and red line. The thin green lines indicate time intervals of 1 second. Note the desynchronization in the EEG beginning from the arrow for the next 1-2 seconds together with a longer lasting decrease in momentarily heart frequency.

According to widely accepted procedures [20-22], we analyzed the maximal amplitudes and latencies of the first negative component (N1), of the second positive component (P2), and we analyzed the area under the curve for the second negative component (N2) in the time range from 250-340 ms. The latter was done since not in all cases we could discern a typical or even a single peak for the component of the AEP. The MMN was measured as the difference curve between the AEP to deviant and parent chords in that time interval (Figure 5). Amplitudes and latencies were compared between parent and deviant stimuli by t-tests (student) and between the groups by one-way ANOVA as well. Separate tests were performed to determine whether the MMN-amplitudes differed for non-musicians and professional musicians as well as for normal hearing musicians and hearing-impaired musicians.

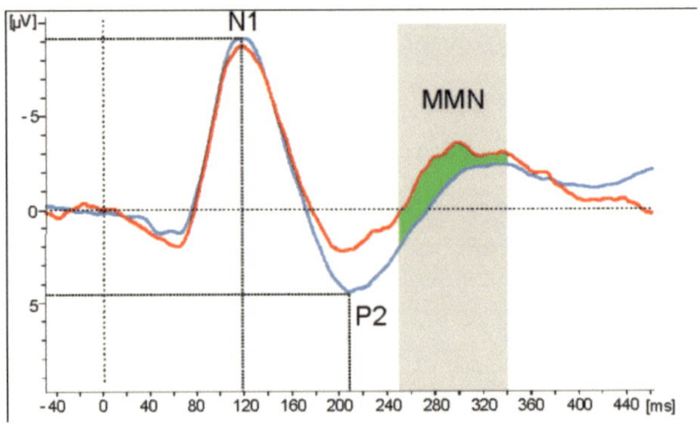

Figure 5. Specimen of a mean auditory evoked potential with labeling of the N1 and P2 components (amplitudes and latencies accentuated with dotted lines). The time interval in which we looked for the MMN is marked in grey, and the MMN is marked in green. The blue curve depicts the mean value to the frequently presented (parent) stimuli, the red one to the infrequently presented (deviant) stimuli.

To assess whether listening to mistuned chords had influence on momentary EEG-activity, we performed a Fast Fourier-Transformation (FFT) with the BrainVision Analyzer 2 in the interstimulus interval to see whether EEG-activity shifted to higher frequencies after mistuned chords. In addition, we analyzed the changes in mean heart rate (average of the heart rate during listening to in-tune music vs. mistuned tones) within the same time interval. A statistical comparison was made by means of the Wilcoxon matched pairs signed-ranks test. Statistical significance was set at 5%. Though we performed the analysis for all EEG electrodes, for better clarity we present here only data from the Cz electrodes.

3. Results

3.1. Amplitudes and latencies of N1 and P2 components of the AEP in normal hearing probands

As can be seen in Figure 6, our presented chords evoked stable and replicable AEP both in non-musicians and in professional musicians that differed only slightly between both groups.

http://dx.doi.org/10.5772/61137

In both groups the presentation of mistuned chords induced larger P2 components than the presentation of normal chords.

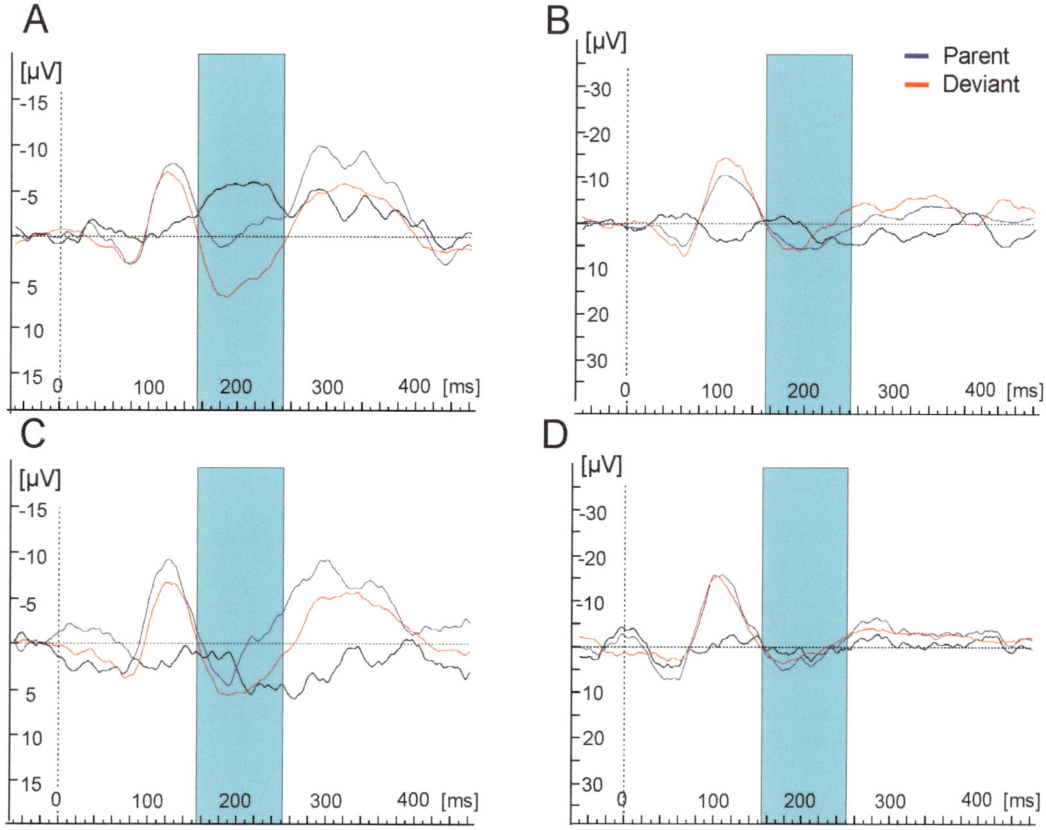

Figure 6. Mean values of AEP evoked by normal or mistuned stimuli in musicians (left diagrams) and in non-musicians (right diagrams). The bluish areas mark the time range in which we analyzed the differences between the AEP. The difference curves are shown in black. The blue lines represent AEP to frequently presented chords, the red lines AEP to the infrequently presented ones. For a better visibility the standard deviations of the curves are omitted. A and B show that normal chords occurred frequently (paradigm 1). C and D show that mistuned chords occurred frequently (paradigm 2). Note the small differences between normal tuned and mistuned chords in non-musicians in diagrams B and D.

The peak of the N1 component was seen at about 128 ms after the stimulus, the peak of the P2 component at about 224 ms after the stimulus. Mean N1 amplitudes amounted to about 7 μV, mean P2 amplitudes to 5 μV. A detailed comparison between the groups of musicians and non-musicians and the three paradigms is given in Figure 7. It should be noted that both C3-major chords resulted in markedly larger areas under the curve both for the N1 and for the P2 components in non-musicians and in musicians. However, the area under the curve of the P2 component was larger when C3-major chords were presented than when C1-major chords were presented.

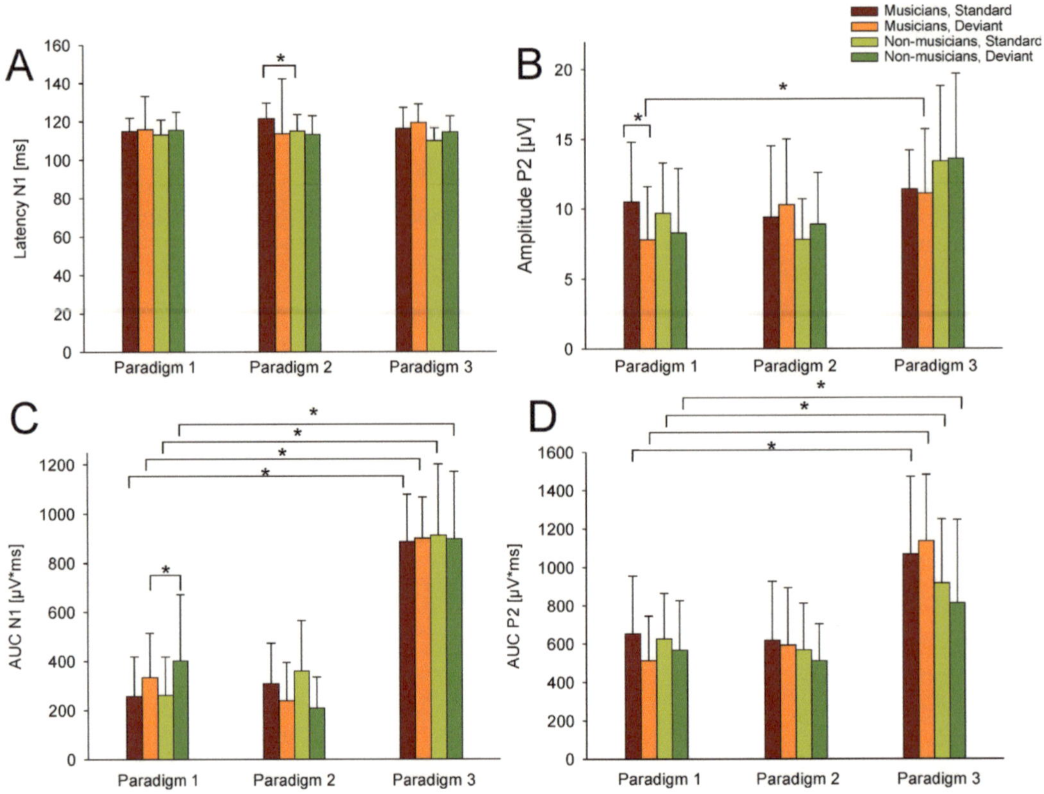

Figure 7. AEP components from normal hearing non-musicians and musicians. The bars give the mean values ± std. dev. The asterisks mark statistically significant differences ($p<0.05$). A) Latency times of the N1 component. B) Amplitudes of the P2 component. C) Areas under the curves of the N1 component. D) Areas under the curve of the P2 component.

Interestingly, the EEG activity differed markedly between both groups when the late components of the AEP were compared that were recorded from the Cz electrode and an activity map was computed by the brain vision software. Though the general pattern was alike, a general higher activity rate was seen in musicians over the temporo-occipital cortex and a lower activity in the vertex area of the brain (Figure 8).

3.2. Amplitudes and latencies of N1 and P2 components of the AEP in hearing-impaired probands

All professional musicians in this group had a hearing loss in the mid- and/or high-frequency range with a mean PTS up to 35 dB SPL. No significant differences were obtained when left and right ears were tested so a preferential side of hearing loss could be excluded. All hearing-impaired industrial workers suffered from hearing loss that was recognized as an occupational disease. The hearing deficit had a similar magnitude as in the hearing-impaired professional musicians and was also found at both ears with a slight but insignificant preference to the left ears (Figure 9).

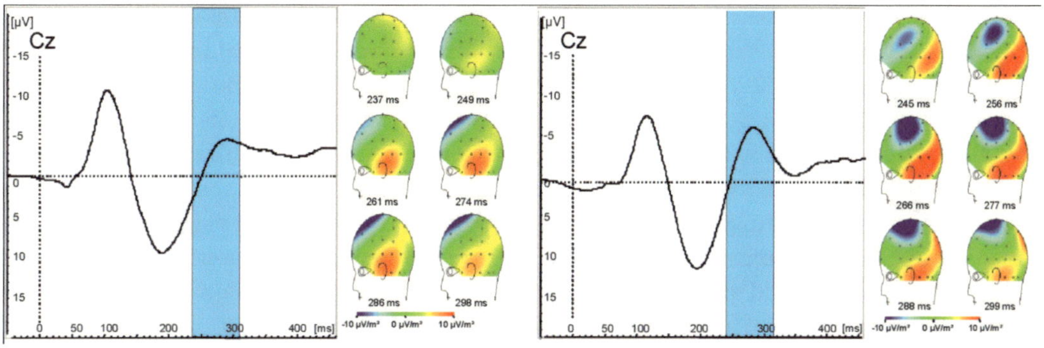

Figure 8. Comparison of cortical EEG activity after stimulation with normal C1-major chords. The AEP curves show the grand mean value from all participants and the activity maps the distribution of cortical activity at different moments after the stimulus in the time range marked in blue. A) Data from normal hearing non-musicians. B) Data from normal hearing musicians.

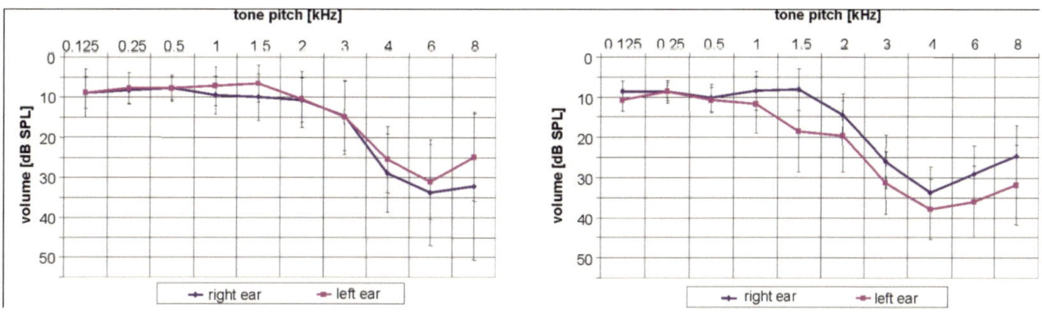

Figure 9. Mean values ± std. dev. of hearing loss in the left and right ears of the 10 hearing-impaired professional musicians (left) and of the 20 hearing-impaired industrial workers (right).

When tested with the auditory stimuli, the parameters of the AEP components differed from the data obtained in normal hearing musicians. The N1 peaks were found earlier (C1 chord 121 ms, C3 chord 109 ms after stimulus) and had larger amplitudes (C1 chord 11 µV, C3 chord 11 µV). The same was seen for the P2 peaks (latency for C1 chords 213 ms, for C3 chords 202 ms; amplitude for C1 chords 5 µV, for C3 chords 8 µV). The latter difference was even significant between C1 chords and C3 chords in this group.

For both stimulus types (normal or mistuned), neither amplitudes nor latencies of the N1 component showed significant differences between non-musicians, normal hearing or hearing-impaired musicians. Responses to parent or deviant stimuli did not differ, regardless whether in-tune or mistuned chords were given as parent stimuli. Similarly, no significant difference existed when comparing the N1 components to the mid-frequency (C1; paradigm 1) or to high-frequency (C3; paradigm 3) stimulation when the chords were mistuned by either 50 cent or by 12 cent.

The workers were first presented the same auditory stimuli as the other participants in this study, i.e., C1-major chords. When analyzing the AEP, we found later N1 amplitudes (peak

134 ms after stimulus) when the paradigm 1 was used, and same latencies as in non-musicians, when the paradigm 2 was used (N1 peak 128 ms after stimulus). The N1 amplitudes ranged from 10 to 12 μV and differed only slightly from those we obtained in non-musicians (Figure 10A and 10B). A similar result was seen when we analyzed the P2 components of the AEP. In this group, the latencies ranged from 228 to 237 ms after stimulus in paradigm 1 and from 218 to 226 ms in paradigm 2 that was later than in musicians, but in the same range as in non-musicians. The P2 amplitudes ranged from 7 to 11 μV and did not differ significantly to the other participants. Both musicians and industrial workers had larger P2 areas under the curve either when the mistuned stimuli were presented rarely in the paradigms 1 (Figure 10C) or often in the paradigms 2 (Figure 10D).

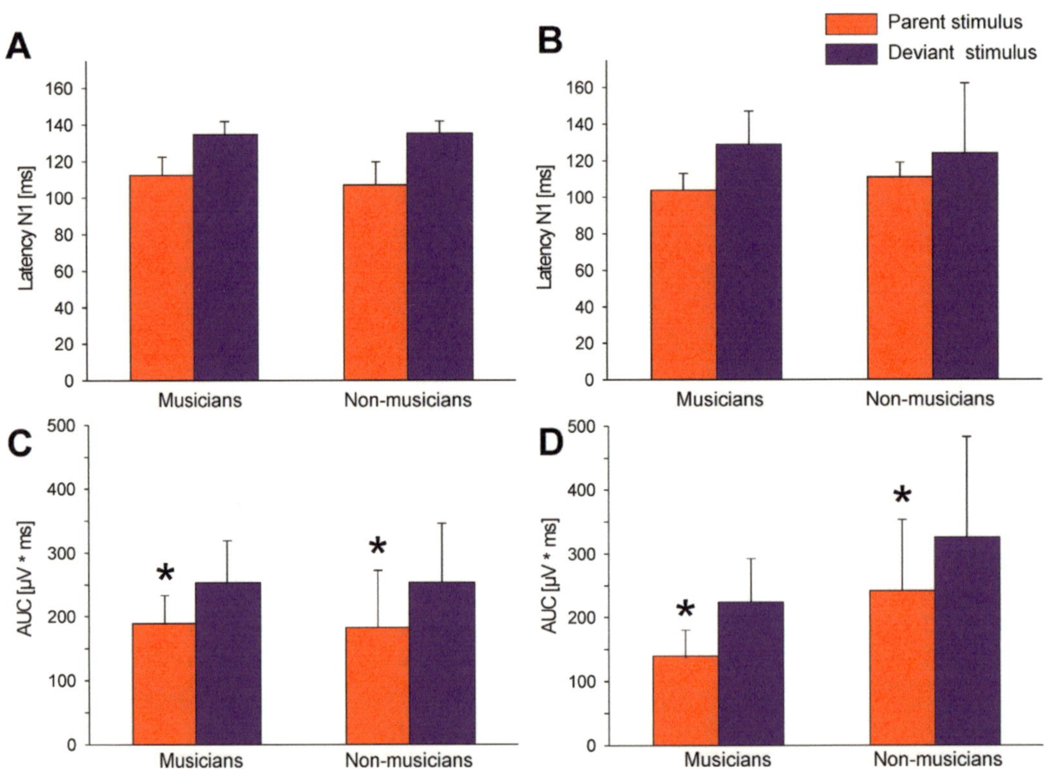

Figure 10. Comparison of amplitudes of the N1 components and of the areas under the curve for the P2 components of the AEP in hearing-impaired musicians and in hearing-impaired industrial workers. Data are presented as mean values ± std. dev. The asterisk marks statistically significant differences ($p<0.05$). A) N1 latencies in paradigm 1. B) N1 latencies in paradigm 2. C) P2 areas under the curve in paradigm 1. D) P2 areas under the curve in paradigm 2.

In a second part of the study, the workers had to listen to machine noise that was either unchanged (parent stimulus) or interrupted/disturbed by short high-pitched whistles. This type of stimulation did not evoke typical AEP, but was used to look for activity changes in the EEG (see below).

3.3. Comparison of the MMN

When interviewed after the series both normal hearing and hearing-impaired musicians complained about the mistuned chords. They told us that they were annoyed at the mistuned chords, but hearing-impaired non-musicians and hearing-impaired industrial workers had not perceived the small differences between the stimuli.

Hearing-impaired musicians were still able to distinguish between in-tune and mistuned chords in both the C1 and in the C3 chords regardless of the degree of mistuning. Their areas under the curve for the MMN were significantly larger when the C1 chords were presented and mistuned stimuli occurred rarely (paradigm 1), which is shown in Figure 11.

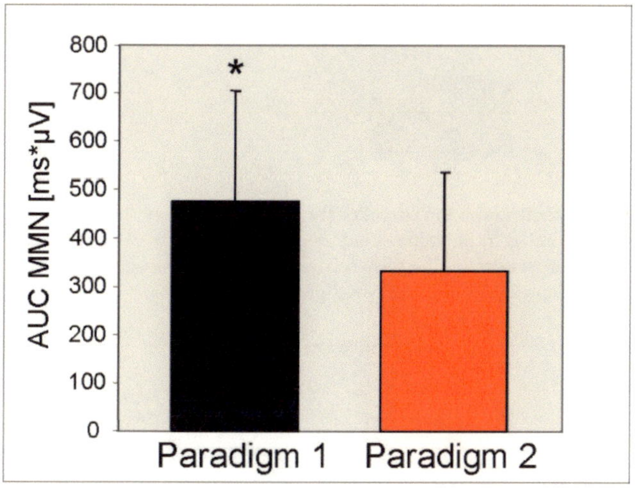

Figure 11. Comparison of areas under the curve for the stimulation with C1 chords in paradigm 1 (black bar) and in paradigm 2 (red bar). Data are presented as mean values ± std. dev. The asterisk marks a significant difference ($p<0.05$).

Independent from hearing impairment, rarely occurring chords (either normal or mistuned) in the musicians group evoked larger areas under the curve for the P2 components (Figure 12).

Interestingly, in hearing-impaired industrial workers, a similar but statistically insignificant difference was seen between the areas under the curve for the P2 component, though the workers told in the interview that they did not observe any differences between the presented chords. This difference was seen both when the mistuned stimulus was presented rarely or often (Figure 13).

The investigation of the MMN curves (AEP to deviant minus AEP to standard stimuli) confirmed differences between non-musicians and both groups of musicians. In normal hearing musicians, the MMN was found in the time range from 180-250 ms after stimulus and a similar, but even longer lasting MMN (up to 300 ms after stimulus), was seen in hearing-impaired musicians. The MMN curves after high-frequency stimulation (C3 chords), however, allowed a clear differentiation between professional musicians and non-musicians. Non-

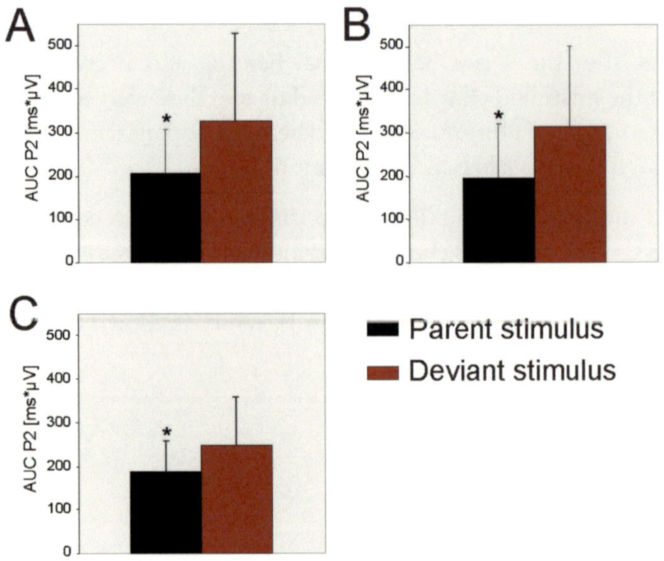

Figure 12. Comparison of the areas under the curve for the P2 components of the AEP in hearing-impaired professional musicians. Data are presented as mean values ± std. dev. The asterisks mark significant differences ($p<0.05$). Black bars show responses to the parent stimuli, the brown bars show the responses to the deviant stimuli. A) C1 chord, paradigm 1. B) C1chord, paradigm 2. C) C3 chord, paradigm 3.

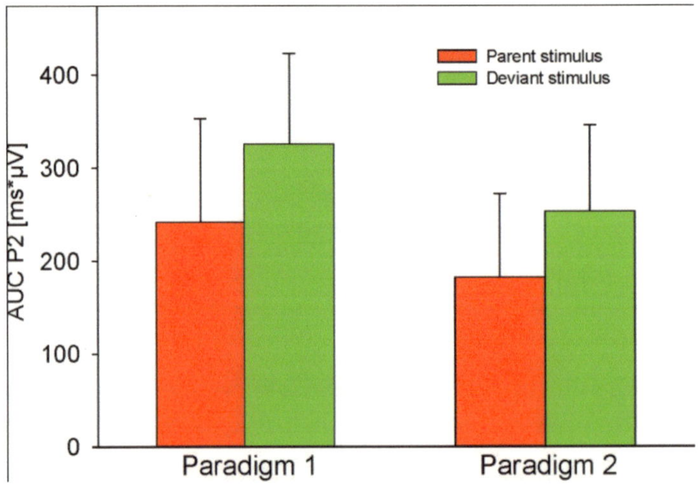

Figure 13. Areas under the curve for the P2 component recorded in hearing-impaired workers. Data are presented as mean values ± std. dev. The red bars show responses to parent stimuli, the green ones to deviant stimuli. A) Presentation in paradigm 1 (mistuned stimuli occur rarely). B) Presentation in paradigm 2 (normal stimuli occur rarely).

musicians had no typical MMN in the observed time range. In normal hearing musicians, this MMN occurred in the range of 250-340 ms after stimulus and a small, but clearly discernable MMN was also found in hearing-impaired musicians. In the latter group, however, the MMN started earlier (220-230 ms after stimulus).

3.4. FFT analysis of the EEG and heart rate analysis

Due to the instructions to the participants (closed eyes, relaxed sitting position, no directed attention to the stimuli), highest spectral power was found in the alpha band, thus confirming that the participants followed the instructions. In both groups of musicians, we found a shift in power density towards higher alpha EEG activity in the interstimulus intervals after presentation of mistuned chords. Such a large shift failed to occur in non-musicians, when the same stimuli were presented. In this group EEG power spectra density was the same, regardless whether in-tune or mistuned chords were presented (Figure 14).

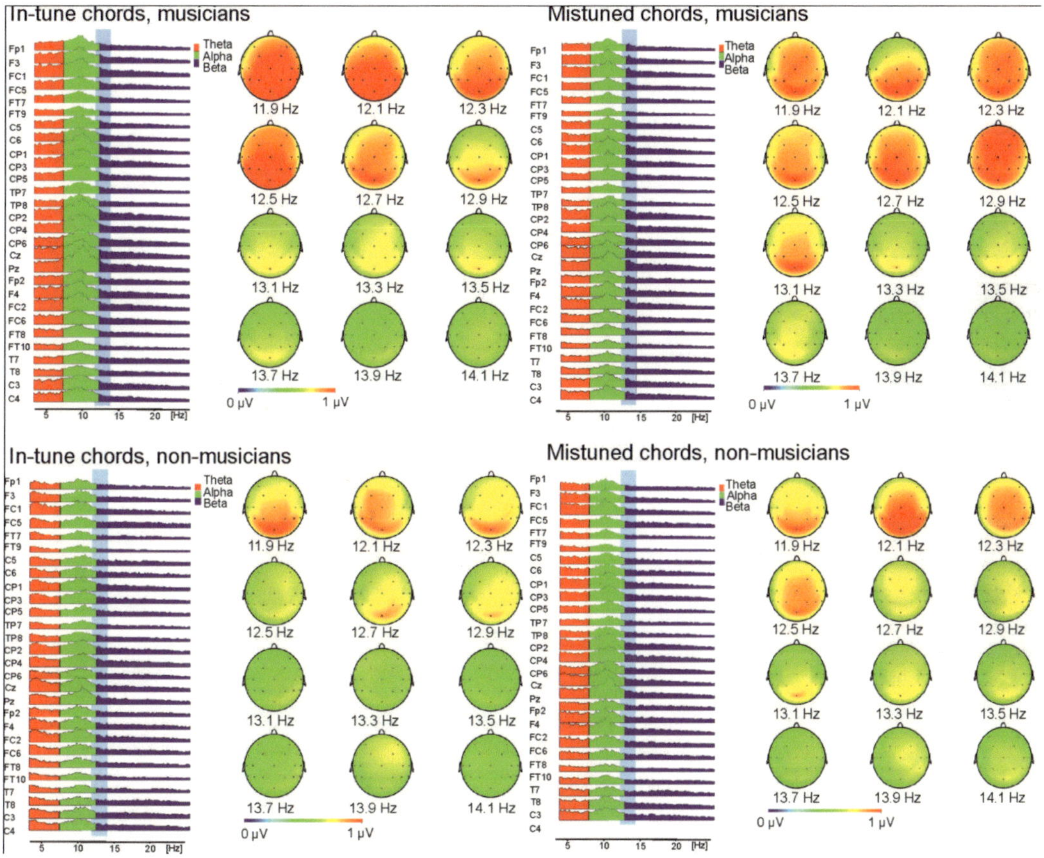

Figure 14. FFT-analysis of the EEG shown as diagrams of regional spectral EEG power and as frequency split maps for musicians (top) and non-musicians (bottom). The light blue bar in the power spectra marks the frequency range that is further analyzed in the frequency split maps. Note the activity shifts towards higher alpha frequencies in musicians when mistuned stimuli were presented. Such a shift failed to occur in non-musicians.

In the same groups we analyzed the heart rates and found a significant increase in mean heart rate in musicians after listening to mistuned chords compared to the resting situation, but no significant differences when comparing resting situation vs. hearing of in-tune chords (resting situation 69.6±12.4 beats per minute, 70.2±12.4 beats per minute after in-tune chords, 71.4±11.5

beats per minute after mistuned chords; n=15; Wilcoxon matched pairs signed-ranks test, p=0.0353). The mean heart frequency, however, did not change in non-musicians (resting situation 60,7±8.1 beats per minute, 60.5±7.5 beats per minute after in-tune chords, 60.8±8.7 beats per minute after mistuned chords; n=10).

Hearing-impaired industrial workers always negated to have noticed the mistuned stimuli, though we had recorded typical MMN to the rare stimulus. In order to present a profession-specific sound to this group, we had used short sequences of the unchanged machine noise and the same noise with high-pitched whistles that sounded like very short pips.

As expected from the pre-trial interviews where the hearing-impaired workers claimed that they easily could discern even one broken bottle in the machine sound, the workers confirmed after the trials that they had heard the rarely occurring disturbed noise samples. In the EEG, the occurrence of these rare stimuli caused a desynchronization lasting for 5-6 seconds (Figure 15).

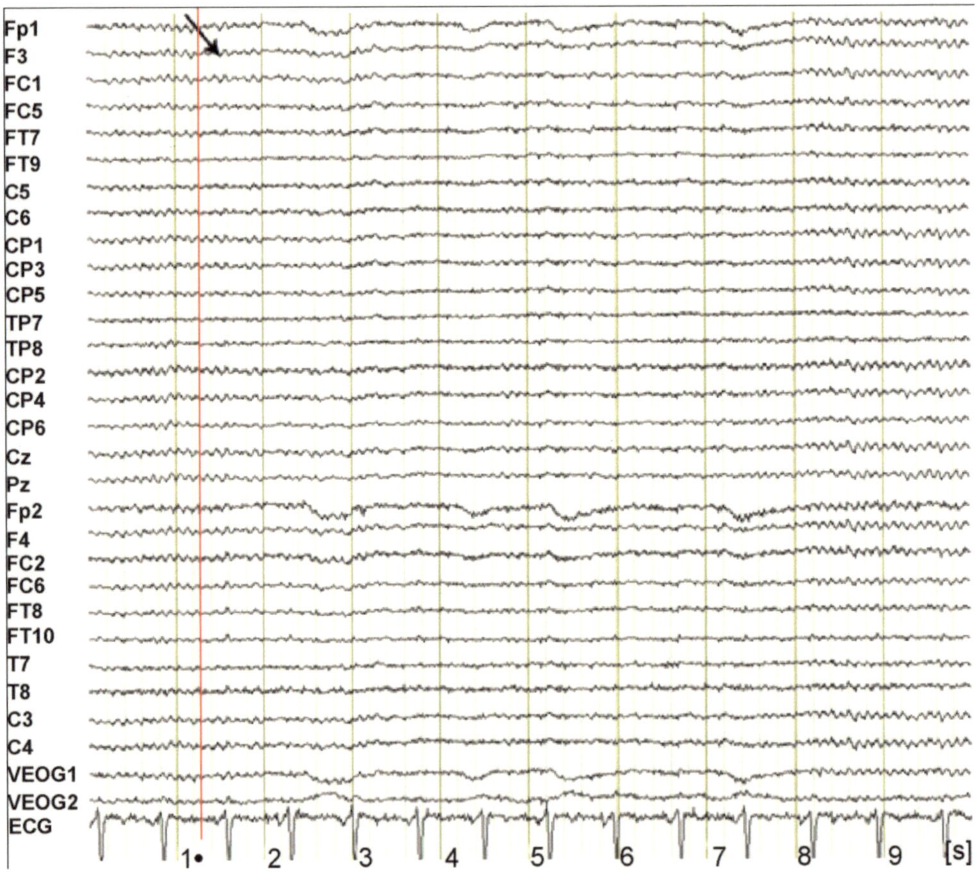

Figure 15. Sample EEG recording from one hearing-impaired industrial worker. The black dot at the bottom marks the presentation of the disturbed machine noise; the onset of the desynchronization in the EEG is marked by an arrow.

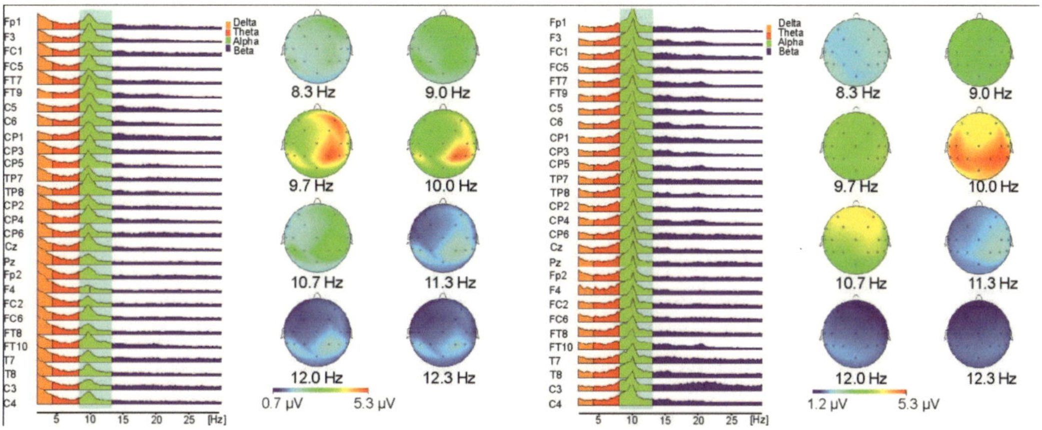

Figure 16. FFT-analysis of the EEG shown as diagrams of regional spectral EEG power and as frequency split maps for normal undisturbed machine noise was presented (left panel), and when the machine noise was disturbed by short pips (right panel). The light blue bar in the power spectra marks the frequency range that is further analyzed in the frequency split maps.

We performed the same FFT-analysis of the EEG in the workers and revealed a shift in the frequency towards higher alpha bands when the disturbed noise was presented (Figure 16). During undisturbed noise the EEG activity had its maximum at 9.7 Hz and was preferentially distributed in the right hemisphere, and only a small area of this hemisphere showed a 10.0 Hz EEG. When we presented the disturbed noise, in a larger area of the brain at both hemispheres a 10.0 Hz EEG and in the frontal parts of the cortex even a 10.7 Hz EEG were observed. The mean EEG frequency increased from 9.2±0.6 Hz during undisturbed noise to 9.4±0.6 Hz during disturbed noise.

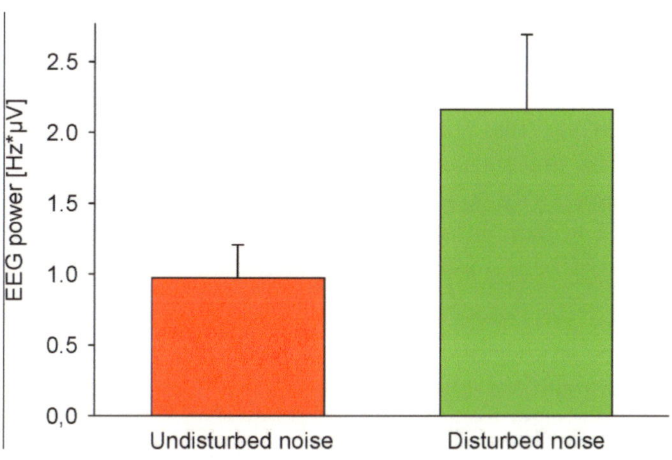

Figure 17. Mean values of EEG power spectra ± std. dev. in hearing-impaired industrial workers when typical machine noise was presented. The red bar shows the data during undisturbed noise; the green one shows the data during disturbed noise.

In addition, we analyzed the power spectra in the frequency range from 12 to 14 Hz at the Cz electrode and found significantly higher regional EEG spectral power in hearing-impaired industrial workers when disturbed machine noise was presented (Figure 17).

4. Discussion

For the first time in this study, profession-specific stimuli were used to assess the effects of hearing deficits in professional musicians and in industrial workers. Here we have shown that parameters of AEP and MMN to mistuned chords differ between musicians and non-musicians, as well as between normal hearing and hearing-impaired musicians, and that components of the AEP and the MMN can be used to differentiate between the three investigated groups. FFT analysis of the EEG in the interstimulus intervals confirmed that mistuned chords caused a state of higher EEG activity only in musicians, regardless of their hearing loss. Another evidence was the occurrence of heart rate changes only in musicians. Therefore we conclude that both perception and processing of musical signals differ between musicians and non-musicians. In hearing-impaired workers, the disturbed machine noise caused a state of higher EEG activity as well.

It is known that complex stimuli such as complex derived words can produce MMN [23]. The stimuli we used were chosen from the typical occupational environment of the professional musician, i.e., musical chords. Complex musical sounds are used to produce MMN, e.g., to compare timbre processing in harmonically rich sounds versus single sinusoidal tones [24]. We had expected that musicians with ongoing musical training over several years have learned to hear and to evaluate these stimuli with their professional memory. Marked differences between tuned and mistuned chords should be recognized easily by musicians, but also by non-musicians. Smaller differences, however, when stimuli were presented in the high-frequency range should be recognized only by musicians. To our knowledge, such a study had not been done before in hearing-impaired musicians.

Intense musical training resulted in an increase in area of primary and secondary auditory cortices [25-27]. In line with this finding, fMRI investigations in musicians revealed a co-activation of both auditory and sensomotor areas in the cortex, thus showing that musical training changes the connectivity and probably also the processing strategies in the brain of musicians [28-30]. Long-term musical training enhances the short-term memory for auditory stimuli and eased behavioral tasks, e.g., detection of deviant tones in a series of auditory stimuli [31].

Our results confirmed the efficacy of comparison of event-related potentials to differentiate between trained musicians and non-musicians [32,33]. The effect of training to induce neural plasticity in the auditory system has been shown in musical conductors compared to non-musicians in a spatial detection task [34], in a pitch detection task [35] or in MMN evoked by variations of complex tone patterns, where long-term musical training modulated the encoding of wrong tones in the right hemisphere of musicians [36]. This is an ongoing process starting in pre-adolescence, since musically trained children had larger MMN to slightly mistuned tones compared to age-matched, non-trained children already at the age of 11, thus confirming that musical training indeed could be responsible for the larger negativity [37]. The cortical plasticity can even be improved, if not only auditory but also somatosensory tasks should be solved, e.g., learning to judge whether music was correctly played versus learning to play an instrument [38]. Interestingly, in hearing-impaired musicians we found clearly distinguishable MMNs, as well as changes in EEG power spectra after presentation of mistuned chords. Even when the stimulus was in the frequency range that was affected by the hearing disability (C3 paradigm), the professional musicians were able to differentiate between in-tune and mistuned chords. However, the normal hearing untrained non-musicians were only able to differentiate to heavily mistuned (50 cent) stimuli, but the hearing impaired did not. The results of interviews confirmed that the mistuned stimuli were recognized both by normal hearing and by hearing-impaired musicians and caused a state of unhappiness.

We could prove this when we tested the hearing-impaired workers with chord stimuli. The workers had similar hearing deficits in a similar frequency range as the hearing professional musicians. The musicians easily recognized the mistuned stimuli and commented on their occurrence in the interviews after the trials, but the workers who never before had heard those stimuli did not. The early AEP components (N1 amplitudes and latencies) did not indicate different processing of the mistuned chords by the workers. The late AEP components (P2 area under the curve and MMN), however, indicated that the mistuned stimuli were sensed and processed differently, even if the person was not aware of this stimulus [39]. Unfortunately, we could not test this phenomenon reversely with the professional musicians, since they refused stimulation with machine noise. We suppose that such unfamiliar stimuli would be difficult to discern by the musicians.

To explain the ability of hearing-impaired musicians to differentiate between "right" and "wrong" tunes several considerations are necessary. We can exclude a significantly varied loudness of the tuned versus the mistuned stimuli. In the group of hearing-impaired musicians, audiological investigations provided evidence for a diminished peripheral input. This impairment might explain the delayed and smaller amplitude of the P2 component as well as the smaller areas under the curve for the N2 component and the smaller resulting MMNs than in normal hearing musicians. Interestingly, the AEP had a similar amplitude and time shape both after stimulation with the high-frequent C3 paradigm and with the mid-frequent C1-major chords, thus confirming that the hearing damage should have affected a larger part of the cochlea. In agreement with a previous study [8], we had instructed the participants to sit relaxed and not to pay attention to the chords. Therefore, we conclude that we were able to record a non-attentional, automatic processing of musical signals. Musicians that were trained to those signals should process this information more effectively [8]. In line with this, musicians were less dependent on the salience of an acoustical environment, but in non-musicians salience had a stronger impact on the processing of complex tone patterns [36]. Assuming that musical training had already caused this effect before hearing impairment started, it is likely that the diminished input could be processed in professional musicians with still higher efficacy than in untrained non-musicians. Another statement in the literature [10] gives support to our interpretation: musical training should result in a more accurate tuning of the frequency-specific neurons in musicians compared to non-musicians. There is indication for a better top-down modulation of auditory processing in trained musicians for both musical sounds and speech [40]. We suppose, therefore, that a better tuning function of the neurons would result in more accurate processing of the rest of a signal when the input is diminished by cochlear damage. In line with this, we found in hearing-impaired musicians significant earlier N1 and P2 components than in hearing-impaired industrial workers when musician-specific chords were used as stimuli.

We conclude that our observed smaller MMNs to mistuned chords in hearing-impaired professional musicians reflect central compensation mechanisms that are able to improve the processing of profession-specific signals, i.e., musical chords. This compensation does not take place in situations of normal life (i.e., without ongoing formal training), e.g., watching TV, using a headphone or cellular phone, or in situations with a loud background that disturbs the incoming signals. In these situations, hearing-impaired musicians complain about the hearing deficit though they are able to play their instruments correctly.

The musicians investigated in our study were interested in learning about hearing damage and the proper use of hearing protectors. Nevertheless, the acceptance of hearing protectors (custom-built ear plugs for specific instruments) among musicians in classical orchestras is very small; more than 90% dislike such devices. Another number has been observed among rock musicians - there is a rate of nearly 50% who accept such hearing protectors [41,42]. Hearing loss among professional musicians in Germany has so far not been accepted as an occupational disease though sound intensities exceed the limits allowed for a working shift in many orchestras [12,43]. The lack of rules to prevent hearing loss in professional classical musicians and the ongoing dispute whether sound exposure during rehearsals or performances is high enough to induce hearing loss hinders the discussion to foster the use of hearing protection in that profession [44-48].

In conclusion, our data indicate that a differentiation between non-musicians and musicians is possible by analyzing AEP components or the MMN when profession-specific stimuli are used. The MMN was still present in hearing-impaired professional musicians, although they had a hearing deficit in the frequency range of the musical stimuli. Probably, the intense musical training has enhanced the processing structures and/or efficacy to evaluate the musical stimulus. A similar result was seen in the workers: ongoing professional training enabled the detection of disturbed machine noise though this group was unable to detect differences in non-trained musical sounds.

To answer the hypotheses postulated at the beginning:

1. Musical chords are a suitable stimulus to evoke stable and replicable AEP both in musicians and in people who are not trained to musical stimuli. AEP evoked by those stimuli can be used to differentiate between trained and untrained persons. Especially the late components of the AEP differ and depend on the learned stimulus. Ongoing professional training to specific sounds is a learning process that is reflected in different sound processing and in the late components of the AEP.

http://dx.doi.org/10.5772/61137

2. After ongoing training to profession-specific sounds, a person is able to notice even small differences of a stimulus, even though the stimulus is presented in a frequency range with impaired hearing function. This phenomenon should be noted when hearing thresholds are measured. A PTS does not always represent an inability to perform a specific (learned) hearing task.
3. The occurrence of differences in the stimuli that is reflected in different parameters of the AEP does not imply an awareness of perception of the stimulus. This is important when foreign stimuli are used and the proband is asked for recognition of different stimuli.

Nomenclature and Abbreviations

AEP; Auditory evoked potential

ANOVA; Analysis of variance

DPOAE; Distortion product otoacoustic emissions

EEG; Electroencephalogram

FFT; Fast Fourier transformation

MMN; Mismatch Negativity

PTS; Permanent threshold shift

TEOAE; Transient-evoked otoacoustic emissions

VEOG; Vertical electrooculogram

Acknowledgements

The study has been supported by a grant of the Berufsgenossenschaft Nahrungsmittel und Gaststätten (Employer's Liability Insurance Association) and by the Kompetenzzentrum für Interdisziplinäre Prävention (KIP) of the Friedrich Schiller University Jena.

Author details

Edeltraut Emmerich, Marcus Engelmann, Melanie Rohmann and Frank Richter*

Institute of Physiology I/Neurophysiology, University Hospital Jena - Friedrich Schiller University, Jena, Germany

References

[1] Näätänen R, Gaillard AWK, Mäntysalo S. Early selective-attention effect on evoked potential reinterpreted. Acta Psychologica. 1978;42:313-329.

[2] Näätänen R, Paavilainen P, Rinne T, Alho K. The mismatch negativity (MMN) in basic research of central auditory processing: A review. Clinical Neurophysiology. 2007;118(12):2544-2590.

[3] Näätänen R, Paavilainen P, Reinikainen K. Do event-related potentials to infrequent decrements in duration of auditory stimuli demonstrate a memory trace in man? Neuroscience Letters. 1989;107(1-3):347-352.

[4] Hari R, Hämäläinen M, Ilmoniemi R, Kaukoranta E, Reinikainen K, Salminen J, Alho K, Näätänen R, Sams M. Responses of the primary auditory cortex to pitch changes in a sequence of tone pips: Neuromagnetic recordings in man. Neuroscience Letters. 1984;50(1-3):127-132.

[5] Näätänen R, Paavilainen P, Alho K, Reinikainen K, Sams M. The mismatch negativity to intensity changes in an auditory stimulus sequence. Electroencephalography & Clinical Neurophysiology. 1987;Suppl. 40:125-131.

[6] Tervaniemi M, Winkler I, Näätänen R. Pre-attentive categorization of sounds by timbre as revealed by event-related potentials. Neuroreport. 1997;8(11):2571-2574.

[7] Rahne T, Plontke SK, Wagner L. Mismatch negativity (MMN) reflects timbre discrimination thresholds in normal-hearing listeners and cochlear implant users. Brain Research. 2014;1586:143-151.

[8] Rüsseler J, Altenmüller E, Nager W, Kohlmetz C, Münte TF. Event-related brain potentials to sound omissions differ in musicians and non-musicians. Neuroscience Letters. 2001;308(1):33-36.

[9] Leino S, Brattico E, Tervaniemi M, Vuust P. Representation of harmony rules in the human brain: Further evidence from event-related potentials. Brain Research. 2007;1142:169-177.

[10] Koelsch S, Schröger E, Tervaniemi M. Superior pre-attentive auditory processing in musicians. Neuroreport. 1999;10(6):1309-1313.

[11] Vuust P, Pallesen KJ, Bailey C, van Zuijen TL, Gjedde A, Roepstorff A, Østergaard L. To musicians, the message is in the meter pre-attentive neuronal responses to incongruent rhythm are left-lateralized in musicians. Neuroimage. 2005;24(2):560-564.

[12] Emmerich E, Rudel L, Richter F. Is the audiologic status of professional musicians a reflection of the noise exposure in classical orchestral music? European Archives of Otorhinolaryngology. 2008;265(7):753-758.

[13] Bormann V, Sust CA, Heinecke-Schmidt R, Fuder G, Lazarus H., editors. Schwerhörigkeit und Sprachkommunikation am Arbeitsplatz. Schriftenreihe der

Bundesanstalt für Arbeitsschutz und Arbeitsmedizin - Fb 1041. Dortmund: Wirtschaftsverlag NW; 2005.

[14] Gentsch G. Differenzierung reiner und verstimmter Akkorde bei hörgeschädigten Berufsmusikern: Eine Analyse akustisch evozierter Potentiale. MD thesis. University Hospital Jena - Friedrich Schiller University; 2010.

[15] Rohmann M. Analyse von akustisch evozierten Potentialen nach reinen und verstimmten Akkorden bei hörgesunden Musikern und Nichtmusikern. MD thesis. University Hospital Jena - Friedrich Schiller University; 2012.

[16] Münte TF, Altenmüller E, Jäncke L. The musician's brain as a model of neuroplasticity. Nature Reviews Neuroscience. 2002;3(6):473-478.

[17] Parbery-Clark A, Anderson S, Kraus N. Musicians change their tune: How hearing loss alters the neural code. Hearing Research. 2013;302:121-131.

[18] Kral A, Eggermont JJ. What's to lose and what's to learn: Development under auditory deprivation, cochlear implants and limits of cortical plasticity. Brain Research Reviews. 2007;56(1):259-269.

[19] Spada D, Verga L, Iadanza A, Tettamanti M, Perani D. The auditory scene: An fMRI study on melody and accompaniment in professional pianists. Neuroimage. 2014;102:764-775.

[20] Koelsch S, Gunter TC, Wittfoth M, Sammler D. Interaction between syntax processing in language and in music: An ERP Study. Journal of Cognitive Neuroscience. 2005;17(10):1565-1577.

[21] Sussman ES, Gumenyuk V. Organization of sequential sounds in auditory memory. Neuroreport. 2005;16(13):1519-1523.

[22] Tata MS, Ward LM. Early phase of spatial mismatch negativity is localized to a posterior "where" auditory pathway. Experimental Brain Research. 2005;167(3): 481-486.

[23] Hanna J, Pulvermuller F. Neurophysiological evidence for whole form retrieval of complex derived words: A mismatch negativity study. Frontiers in Human Neuroscience. 2014;8:886.

[24] Christman, CA, Lachmann T, Berti S. Earlier timbre processing of instrumental tones compared to equally complex spectrally rotated sounds as revealed by the mismatch negativity. Neuroscience Letters. 2014;581:115-119.

[25] Altenmüller E. Brain electrical correlates of cerebral music processing in the human. European Archives of Psychiatry and Neurological Sciences. 1986;235(6):342-354.

[26] Ragert P, Schmidt A, Altenmüller E, Dinse HR. Superior tactile performance and learning in professional pianists: Evidence for meta-plasticity in musicians. European Journal of Neuroscience. 2004;19(2):473-478.

[27] Koelsch S. Brain correlates of music-evoked emotions. Nature Reviews Neuroscience. 2014;15(3):170-180.

[28] Gaser C, Schlaug G. Brain structures differ between musicians and non-musicians. The Journal of Neuroscience. 2003;23(27):9240-9245.

[29] Lotze M, Scheler G, Tan HR, Braun C, Birbaumer N, The musician's brain: Functional imaging of amateurs and professionals during performance and imagery. Neuroimage. 2003;20(3):1817-1829.

[30] Schlaug G, Norton A, Overy K, Winner E. Effects of music training on the child's brain and cognitive development. Annals of the New York Academy of Sciences. 2005;1060:219-230.

[31] Boh B, Herholz SC, Lappe C, Pantev C. Processing of complex auditory patterns in musicians and nonmusicians. PLoS One. 2011;6(7):e21458.

[32] Münte TF, Nager W, Beiss T, Schroeder C, Altenmüller E. Specialization of the specialized: Electrophysiological investigations in professional musicians. Annals of the New York Academy of Sciences. 2003;999:131-139.

[33] Paraskevopoulos E, Kuchenbuch A, Herholz SC, Pantev C. Statistical learning effects in musicians and non-musicians: An MEG study. Neuropsychologia. 2012;50(2): 341-349.

[34] Münte TF, Kohlmetz C, Nager W, Altenmüller E. Neuroperception. Superior auditory spatial tuning in conductors. Nature. 2001;409(6820):580.

[35] Münte TF, Nager W, Rosenthal O, Johannes S, Altenmüller E. Attention to pitch in musicians and non-musicians: An event-related brain potential study. In: Nakada T. (ed.) Integrated Human Brain Science. Amsterdam: Elsevier; 2000. p. 389-398.

[36] Kuchenbuch A, Paraskevopoulos E, Herholz SC, Pantev C. Effects of musical training and event probabilities on encoding of complex tone patterns. BMC Neuroscience. 2013;14:51.

[37] Putkinen V, Tervaniemi M, Saarkivi K, de Vent N, Huotilainen M. Investigating the effects of musical training on functional brain development with a novel Melodic MMN paradigm. Neurobiology of Learning and Memory. 2014;110:8-15.

[38] Pantev C, Lappe C, Herholz SC, Trainor L. Auditory-somatosensory integration and cortical plasticity in musical training. Annals of the New York Academy of Sciences. 2009;1169:143-150.

[39] Engelmann M. Untersuchungen von Komponenten akustisch evozierter Potentiale an schwerhörigen Industriearbeitern. MD thesis. University Hospital Jena - Friedrich Schiller University; 2012.

[40] Tervaniemi M, Kruck S, De Baene W, Schroger E, Alter K.Friederici AD. Top-down modulation of auditory processing: Effects of sound context, musical expertise and attentional focus. European Journal of Neuroscience. 2009;30(8):1636-1642.

[41] Axelsson A, Eliasson A, Israelsson B. Hearing in pop/rock musicians: A follow-up study. Ear and Hearing. 1995;16(3):245-253.

[42] Schmuziger N, Patscheke J, Probst R. Hearing in nonprofessional pop/rock musicians. Ear and Hearing. 2006;27(4):321-330.

[43] Emmerich E, Richter F, Hagner H, Giessler F, Gehrlein S, Dieroff HG. Effects of discotheque music on audiometric results and central acoustic evoked neuromagnetic responses. International Tinnitus Journal. 2002;8(1):13-19.

[44] Toppila E, Koskinen H, Pyykkö I. Hearing loss among classical-orchestra musicians. Noise & Health. 2011;13(50):45-50.

[45] O'Brien I, Driscoll T, Ackermann B. Hearing conservation and noise management practices in professional orchestras. Journal of Occupational and Environmental Hygiene. 2012; 9(10):602-608.

[46] Schmidt JH, Pedersen ER, Paarup HM, Christensen-Dalsgaard J, Andersen T, Poulsen T, Bælum J. Hearing loss in relation to sound exposure of professional symphony orchestra musicians. Ear and Hearing. 2014;35(4):448-60.

[47] Schink T, Kreutz G, Busch V, Pigeot I, Ahrens W. Incidence and relative risk of hearing disorders in professional musicians. Occupational & Environmental Medicine. 2014;71(7):472-476.

[48] Raymond DM 3rd, Romeo JH, Kumke KV. A pilot study of occupational injury and illness experienced by classical musicians. Workplace Health & Safety. 2012;60(1): 19-24.

Section 4

Hearing Loss and Tinnitus

Chapter 8

A Combination of EGb 761 and Soft Laser Therapy in Chronic Tinnitus

Klára Procházková, Ivan Šejna, Petr Schalek, Jozef Rosina and Aleš Hahn

Additional information is available at the end of the chapter

http://dx.doi.org/10.5772/61740

Abstract

Objective: We aimed to verify the therapeutic effect of soft laser in a combination with Ginkgo biloba extract EGb 761 in patients suffering from chronic tinnitus.

Background data: Tinnitus is described as an illusory sound perceived by the patient when there is no corresponding source of this sound outside. Tinnitus may signify a disturbance of peripheral or central part of hearing system. Beside the hearing system, there might be an utterly different etiology of tinnitus. Cardiovascular, musculoskeletal, mental, and other disorders can contribute to tinnitus formation as well. Due to these multiple etiologic factors the treatment is very difficult.

Studies analyzing biological effects of EGb 761 and laser suggest their use in tinnitus treatment. However, clinical study results are very variable, which makes their general use more controversial.

Methods: We conducted a simple prospective study including 420 patients suffering from chronic tinnitus (duration 3 months to 40 years; 7.7 years mean value; SD 7.8). A soft laser BTL-10 type was used with an 830 nm / 200 mV probe, at an energy density of 50 J/cm^2, applied with transmastoidal and transmeatal approach in a continuous and pulse beam, after 3 weeks of oral use of EGb 761. The therapeutic effect was evaluated by tinnitus intensity and frequency determination (tinnitus masking) and by the subjective rating on visual analogue scale (VAS) with 0 - 10 points.

Results: Among the 420 patients, 238 (56, 7%) achieved improvement in the tinnitus masking, the average improvement in terms of intensity was found to be 30dB. Hundred and ninety-six patients (46, 7%) recorded improvement on VAS. The objective and subjective evaluation coincided in 79% of cases.

Conclusion: Compared to the outcomes of other studies, our findings reveal a relatively higher percentage of positive changes regarding the tinnitus status and greater congruence of objective (audiometric) and subjective (VAS) results.

Keywords: Tinnitus, EGb 761, laser

1. Introduction

Tinnitus is described as an illusory sound perceived by the patient when there is no corresponding source of this sound outside. Tinnitus is present in 5 - 15% of the population and in 70% of patients with hearing disturbances. Tinnitus may signify a disturbance of the peripheral or central part of the hearing system. Beside the hearing system, there are more possible causes of tinnitus - cardiovascular, musculoskeletal, metabolic, and endocrine dysfunctions (dyslipidemia, thyroid dysfunction, diabetes mellitus), and stress and mental disorders might contribute to tinnitus formation as well. Despite the diagnostic tools we have (audiometry, tinnitus masking), the exact cause often remains unrevealed. Various origins of tinnitus make the treatment very difficult and challenging as well, knowing that tinnitus itself can cause another mental and social troubles.

There are numerous chronic tinnitus treatment methods such as pharmacotherapy, physiotherapy, psychotherapy, surgery, etc., which concentrate on the tinnitus intensity reduction and patient's life quality enhancement. Unfortunately, the therapy effect is quite poor in the majority of cases, so alternative modalities of treatment are often introduced. [1] In chronic tinnitus patients, complete disparition of tinnitus arrives very rarely. The number of completely cured patients is not statistically significant.

The therapy is targeted to reducing the tinnitus sensation. We evaluate subjective feelings concerning annoyance and loudness of tinnitus described by means of visual analogue scale (VAS 0-10) and objective measurements of the frequency and intensity of tinnitus.

For better tinnitus control, a combination of treatment methods were inducted. The dual approach of Ginkgo biloba extract (EGb 761) and soft laser therapy belongs to various combined methods.

EGb 761 is a standardized extract containing 24% flavonoids, 7% proanthocyanidins, and 6% terpenoids. [2] It has a polymodal effect on the cell and tissue metabolism. The flavonoids are mainly responsible for antioxidant actions while diminishing the free radical damage. [3, 4, 5, 6] The terpenoid fraction contains Ginkolide B which is a potent platelet-activating factor (PAF) receptor antagonist. [7] EGb 761 is also a vasodilator. For hundreds of years the Ginkgo biloba extract was used for the treatment of respiratory disorders. [8] Some studies deny the therapeutic effect of Egb 761 in tinnitus, [2] while others encourage its use. [9]

Laser devices generate electromagnetic radiation with only one wave length. In the biological tissue, the laser light beams exert analgesic, anti-inflammatory, stimulation, thermal, and photochemical effect. The concentrated radiation reduces the irritability of the peripheral nervous system, activates polymorphous cells, monocytes, granulocytes, and fibroblasts, activates respiration chain enzymes, and amplifies anti-oxidative effects in the mitochondria. The laser radiation intensifies metabolism in targeted tissues and cells. They gain additional energy, they can regenerate faster, and their mechanisms of protection are amplified. [10]

In the field of otoneurology, the red light spectrum lasers are the optimal. Thus, the effect we expect is mainly founded on the support of cellular oxidative processes and cell metabolism stimulation.

For the treatment of tinnitus, low level laser therapy (soft laser therapy) has been used since the early 1990s'. Studies concerning the evaluation of its therapeutic possibilities and achievements followed soon after. For both single therapy by the soft laser [11, 12, 13] and combined therapy by the soft laser with EGb 761, the results have been discouraging. [14] However, recent researches show more promising results. [15, 16, 17, 18, 19, 20] This mismatch of findings can be clarified by different researchers' approaches, which concern the design of the study, physical parameters of the laser beam, topography of the radiated region, and duration and schedule of the laser therapy. Results from more recent surveys [16, 17] are validated and confirmed by functional magnetic resonance and dosimetric studies.

This study follows our former publication, [21] whereas now involving more patients.

2. Materials and methods

At our ENT Clinic of the Third Medical Faculty, Charles University in Prague, we conducted a simple prospective study including 420 patients with chronic maskable tinnitus between years 1998 and 2006. Two hundred women and 220 men were enrolled, and the mean age of patients was 53.7 years (16 - 77 years). The onset of tinnitus was 3 months to 40 years (mean time of onset 7.7 years) (Table 1).

420 patients (200 women and 220 men)		
Age	– group:	16–77 years (53.7 mean; SD = 14.2)
	– women:	16–77 years (54.1 mean; SD = 14.1)
	– men:	16–77 years (53.3 mean; SD = 14.2)
Tinnitus duration	– group:	0.25–40 years (7.7 mean; SD = 7.8)
	– women:	0.50–32 years (7.8 mean; SD = 7.9)
	– men:	0.25–40 years (7.6 mean; SD = 7.7)

Table 1. Study cohort, demography

In the exclusion criteria otosclerosis, vestibular neurinoma, acute labyrinthine disease, serius cervical spine disorders, and serious or non-compensated metabolic disorders were comprehended.

According to the flow chart of the study, we performed thorough history taking, complex ENT examination, audiologic tests (pure tone audiometry, speech audiometry, if necessary objective audiometry as well), tinnitus intensity (dB), and frequency (Hz) determination. The subjective loudness sensation and annoyance were also recorded on visual analogue scale (0-10 points).

Three weeks before the laser therapy started, patients were instructed to take EGb 761 commercial preparations (Tanakan 80 mg or Tebokan 80 mg, in the form of tablet or drops), three times a day by peroral route of administration. The soft laser therapy followed, using BTL-10 laser device. Patients were scheduled for 10 sessions of laser therapy in at least three weeks, each session lasting 10 minutes. The parameters of the probe were adjusted for 830 nm/ 200 mV, at an energy density 50 J/cm^2. Initially a continuous beam followed by the pulse beam were applied, while the probe was targeted to the mastoid process and external auditory canal (aiming to cochlea).

3. Results

As to evaluate the changes of tinnitus, both subjective and objective methods were employed: tinnitus intensity and frequency determination (tinnitus masking) and rating on visual analogue scale (VAS). According to VAS, at least one point less was considered as an improvement.

In terms of audiometric changes, the average intensity improvement was found to be 30 dB (range 10-50 dB). One patient described complete disappearance of tinnitus, and one patient noted worsening of his tinnitus by 10 dB. Tinnitus intensity improved by 10 dB in 31 patients, by 20 dB in 73 patients, by 30 dB in 48 patients, by 40 dB in 38 patients, and eventually by 50 dB in 48 patients. The total number of improved cases equals to 238 (Table 2).

Change	Count	%
by 10 dB	31	13.0
by 20 dB	73	30.6
by 30 dB	48	20.2
by 40 dB	38	16.0
by 50 dB	48	20.2
Σ	238	100.0

Table 2. Objective changes in tinnitus masking

Two hundred and thirty-eight cases (56.7 %) achieved improvement in the tinnitus masking, and in 182 cases (43, 7 %) tinnitus masking remained the same. Subjective relief from tinnitus, recorded by VAS questionnaire, was noted in 196 cases (46.7 %) (Table 3). An interesting observation was made in one female patient with objective improvement of 50 dB and no subjective relief from tinnitus.

Objective parameters		
Audiogram confirming improvement	238 patients	56.7%
Audiogram with no change	182 patients	43.3%
Subjective improvement	196 patients	46.7%

Table 3. Improvement rate

The correlation of subjective and objective measurements was following: in 79% of findings total accord was found (conformity of audiogram and VAS questionnaire), in 11% of cases no subjective improvement was reported in patients with objective audiometrical improvement, and in the remaining 10% of cases, subjective relief from tinnitus was not supported by any objective finding in audiogram (Table 4).

Correlation	Number of patients	%
Conformance of audiogram and VAS	332	79
Audiogram improvement, no VAS change	46	11
VAS improvement, no audiogram change	42	10
$\sum$	420	100

Table 4. Correlation of subjective and objective evaluation

4. Discussion

For the tinnitus evaluation, we can never rely solely on the objective measurement tools. Many relevant factors cannot be measured, but only perceived by the patients. Tinnitus is a very subjective sound sensation, and each person feels it in his own individual way. Hence, the subjective assessment is for us as significant as objective audiometric tests. In our study, regardless the audiometric results, 46.7% of patients described a certain level of relief. The objective tests revealed that an even higher number - 56.7% - of patients displayed improvement with a relatively high mean value of 30dB. Audiometric intensity determination approved the patients' subjective records in 79% of cases, which indicates the relevance of both methods.

The study results are in accord with our everyday experience, when tinnitus intensity determination (tinnitus masking) changes are not always perceived the same way by the patient. In our study cohort 10% of patients reported diminished tinnitus perception, although the audiometric tests showed no change. This might be explicated by the placebo effect. Contrariwise, 11% of the cases were not aware of their "audiologic improvement," which is a routinely described phenomenon of central processing or imprinting of tinnitus. [22, 23]

The therapy was supported well, no serious adverse events were reported, but some patients complained of the laser's thermal effect though.

In comparison to other researches concentrating on soft laser therapy in chronic tinnitus, Shiomi et al. [11] conducted a similar design study but with no premedication by EGb 761.

Finally, he declared similar results in chronic tinnitus patients as we did. In a double-blind randomized study of Gungor et al. [18] who also used laser therapy alone (power of 5 mW, 650 nm wavelength, 15 minutes for one session), the results were similar as in our study. However, Rogowski et al. [13] and Partheniadis-Stumpf et al. [14] found out rather negative outcomes. Such a difference could be explained by different laser parameters and different number of patients in study groups. Compared to the German study, [14] we applied Egb 761 perorally three weeks before the laser therapy, expecting accentuation of the nootropic effect with a longer time of administration, while Partheniadis-Stumpf et al. [14] applied Egb 761 intravenously directly before each laser session.

5. Conclusion

Patients suffering from chronic tinnitus often try numerous therapeutic modalities in a search for alleviation of the stress and annoyance caused by their illness. According to our study results, a combination of Egb 761 and soft laser therapy can be recommended as a safe and suitable modality in the treatment of chronic maskable tinnitus.

6. Disclosure statement

This manuscript has never been submitted for a publication. It is related to, and might be considered as an extension of a previous work, which has been published as:

Hahn, A., Schalek, P., Šejna, I., Rosina, J. (2012). Combined tinnitus therapy with laser and EGb 761: further experiences. Int. Tinnitus J. 17 (1), 50-53

The authors deny any possible conflict of interest related to individual authors' commitments, project support or financial relationships of the authors.

"No competing financial interests exist."

Author details

Klára Procházková[1*], Ivan Šejna[1], Petr Schalek[1], Jozef Rosina[2] and Aleš Hahn[1]

*Address all correspondence to: klara.prochazkova@gmail.com

1 Department of Otorhinolaryngology of the Third Faculty of Medicine, Charles University Prague, Czech Republic

2 Department of Medical Biophysics and Informatics of the Third Faculty of Medicine, Charles University Prague, Czech Republic

http://dx.doi.org/10.5772/61740

References

[1] Meehan, T., Eisenhut, M., Stephens, D. (2004). A review of alternative treatments for tinnitus. Audiol Med. 2, 74–82.

[2] Smith, P.F., Yiwen Zheng, Darlington, C. L. (2005). Ginkgo biloba extracts for tinnitus: More hype than hope? J Ethnopharmacol, 100, 1–2, 95–99.

[3] Maitra, I., Marcocci, L., Droy-Lefax, M.L., Packer, L. (1995). Peroxyl radical scavenging activity of Ginkgo biloba Extract KGB 761. Biochem Pharm. 49, 1649-1655.

[4] Pincemail, J., Deby, C. (1986). Properrietes antiradicalaires de l'extrait de Ginkgo biloba. Presse Med. 15, 1475-1479.

[5] Artmann, G.M., Schikarski, C. (1993). Ginkgo biloba Extract (EGb 761) protects red blood cells from oxidative damage. Clin. Hemorheol. 74-82.

[6] Kose, K., Dogan, P. (1995). Comparison of the antioxidant effect of the Ginkgo biloba extract (EGb 761) with those of water-soluble and lipid-soluble antioxidants. J Int Med Res. 23, 9-18.

[7] Braquet, P.G., Spinnewyn, B., Braquet, M. et al. (1985). BN 52021 and related compounds a new series of highly specific PAF-acether antagonists isolated from Ginkgo biloba. Blood Vessels 16, 558-572.

[8] Kleijnen, J., Knipschild, P. (1992). Ginkgo biloba. Lancet 340, 1136-1139.

[9] Schneider, D., Schneider, L., Shulman, A., Claussen, C.F., Just, E., Koltchev, C., Kersebaum, M., Dehler, R., Goldstein, B., Claussen, E., (2000) Ginkgo biloba (Rokan) therapy in tinnitus patients and measurable interactions between tinnitus and vestibular disturbances. Int Tinnitus J. 6, 56–62.

[10] Chomete, G., Auriol, M., Zeitoun, R. (1987). Effect of the soft laser on gingival tissue. I-Effect on fibroblasts. Histoenzymology and electron microscopy study. J Biol Buccale 15(1), 45-49.

[11] Shiomi. Y., Takahashi, H., Honjo, I. et al. (1997). Efficacy of transmeatal low power laser irradiation on tinnitus: a preliminary report. Auris Nasus Larynx 24(1), 39-42.

[12] Mirz, F., Zachariae, R., Andersen, S.E., Nielsen, S.E. et al. (1999). The low-power laser in the treatment of tinnitus. Clin Otolaryngol. 24(4), 346-354.

[13] Rogowski, M., Mnich, S., Gindzienska, E. et al. (1999). Low power laser in the treatment of tinnitus-a placebo-controlled study. Otolaryngol Pol. 53(3), 315-320.

[14] Partheniadis-Stumpf, M., Maurer, J., Mann, W. (1993). Soft laser therapy in combination with tebonin i.v. in tinnitus. Laryngorhinootologie 72(1), 28-31.

[15] Tauber, S., Baumgartner, R., Schorn, K., Beyer, W. (2001). Lightdosimetric quantitative analysis of the human petrous bone: experimental study for laser irradiation of the cochlea. Lasers Surg Med. 28(1), 18-26.

[16] Tauber, S., Schorn, K., Beyer, W., Baumgartner, R. (2003). Transmeatal cochlear laser (TCL) treatment of cochlear dysfunction: a feasibility study for chronic tinnitus. Lasers Med Sci. 18(3), 154-161.

[17] Siedentopf, C.M., Ischebeck, A., Haala, I.A. et al. (2007). Neural correlates of transmeatal cochlear laser (TCL) stimulation in healthy human subjects. Neurosci. Lett. 411(3), 189-193.

[18] Gungor, A., Dogru, S., Cincik, H., Erkul, E., Poyrazoglu, E. (2007). Effectiveness of transmeatal low power laser irradiation for chronic tinnitus. J Laryngol Otol. 12, 1-5.

[19] Salahaldin, A. H., Abdulhadi, K., Najjar, N., Bener, A. (2012). Low-level laser therapy in patients with complaints of tinnitus: a clinical study. ISRN, Otolaryngol, Article ID 132060.

[20] Okhovat, A., Nezamoddin, B., Okhovat, H., Malekpour, A., Abtahi, H. (2011). Low-level laser for treatment of tinnitus: a self-controlled clinical trial. J Res Med Sci 16(1), 33-38.

[21] Hahn, A., Schalek, P., Šejna, I., Rosina, J. (2012). Combined tinnitus therapy with laser and EGb 761: further experiences. Int Tinnitus J. 17(1), 50-53.

[22] Shulman, A., Goldstein, B. (2006). Tinnitus dyssynchrony-synchrony theory: a translational concept for diagnosis and treatment. Int Tinnitus J. 12(2), 101-114.

[23] Jastreboff, P.J., Hazell, J.W.P. (1993). A neurophysiological approach to tinnitus: clinical implications. Br J Audiol. 27, 7-17.

Section 5

Hearing Screening

Chapter 9

Technological Advances in Universal Neonatal Hearing Screening (UNHS)

Stavros Hatzopoulos, Henryk Skarzynski and Piotr H Skarzynski

Additional information is available at the end of the chapter

http://dx.doi.org/10.5772/61178

Abstract

Within the last decade, numerous new challenges have appeared in the UNHS arena, such as (i) the need to validate the automated OAE/ABR screeners; (ii) the need to qualify the responses from the automated devices; (iii) the need to obtain additional information (i.e., hearing threshold) for the subject under assessment, in a short period of time; (iv) and the need to integrate numerous measurements in a single portable automated device. To respond to these clinical demands, several new methodologies have been introduced to the UNHS clinical practice. In this context, the aim of this chapter is to provide information on these new technological trends.

Keywords: Automated otoacoustic emissions (AOAE), automated auditory brainstem response (AABR), wideband reflectance, middle ear power analysis, neonatal hearing screening, auditory state steady response, hearing threshold

1. Introduction

Otoacoustic emissions (OAEs) or cochlear echoes is a term coined by David Kemp in 1978 [1], describing the transient responses from the inner ear, upon its stimulation by an acoustic click stimulus. During the last 20 years, OAE protocols have been used in many areas of audiology and hearing science [2]. The most significant contribution of OAEs is in the area of universal neonatal hearing screening (UNHS).

While the main objective of neonatal hearing screening (NHS) is the identification of infants with a hearing deficit (≥30 dB HL), the objectives of a UNHS program have a broader vision. Two important phases are considered: (i) the identification of infants with mild and moderate hearing deficits and (ii) an intervention in terms of hearing improvement (hearing aids and cochlear implants) and neural rehabilitation, aiming at the restoration of hearing and the normalization of the quality of life of the young patient.

Within the last decade, numerous new challenges have appeared in the UNHS arena, such as (i) the need to validate the automated OAE/ABR screeners; (ii) the need to qualify the responses from the automated devices; (iii) the need to obtain additional information (i.e., hearing threshold) for the subject under assessment, in a short period of time; and (iv) the need to integrate numerous measurements in a single portable automated device. To respond to these clinical demands, several new methodologies have been introduced to the UNHS clinical practice. In this context, the aim of this chapter is to provide information on these new technological trends.

2. Automated auditory brainstem responses

In the early 2002, the first fourth-generation OAE devices appeared in the market and offered the possibility to integrate information from different testing protocols such as automated OAE (AOAE) and automated ABR (AABR) responses. The combined screening protocols (AOAE + AABR) targeted the identification of auditory neuropathy, most prevalent in the neonatal intensive care (NICU) environment.

With the introduction of the AABR protocols in the NHS programs, several issues became evident, and among those questions related to screening times and screening costs. The latter is outside the objectives of this paper and will not be addressed. A previous study of our group, in the context of the regional NHS project CHEAP in Emilia-Romagna, Italy [3], provided evidence suggesting that in terms of time-requirements, portable ABR (Audioscreener, Viasys; Accuscreen, GN-Otometrics; Algo 3i, Natus) and OAE devices were converging to the same time values. Data from the above study suggested that (i) the average time for AOAE responses is less than 10 s in a cooperative subject and less that 120 s (2 min) in non-cooperative subjects and (ii) the average AABR test times were less than 120 s, while longer times (600 s per ear) were required for uncooperative subjects. The placement of the AABR electrodes might be a complicated process, especially when highly skin impedances (caused by excessive lipid layers) are encountered. In these cases, the AABR algorithms tend to oversample in order to derive a coherent signal, and as a result, the testing times are significantly prolonged.

A combined two-stage approach (i.e., AOAE + AABR) eliminates the risk of not identifying infants with auditory neuropathy and assures that the screening sensitivity is high. Contrary to this hypothesis, data from a large-scale American study by White et al. [4] suggest that this is not always the case. From 86,634 screened infants, using a two-stage OAE/A-ABR protocol, 23% would have passed the AABR.

Another interesting development in the ABR/AABR area is in the area of the evoking stimulus. Traditionally, ABR and AABR protocols use click stimuli to synchronize as many neural fibers as possible and to obtain an ABR response of large amplitude with less sweeps. Recently, chirp stimuli have been used to optimize the ABR/AABR responses. According to Kristensen and

http://dx.doi.org/10.5772/61178

Elberling [5], "Upward chirps are often designed to compensate for the cochlear traveling wave delay which is regarded as independent of stimulation level. A chirp based on a traveling wave model is therefore referred to as a level-independent chirp. Another compensation strategy, for instance based on frequency-specific auditory brainstem response (ABR) latencies, results in a chirp that changes with stimulation level and is therefore referred to as a level-dependent chirp. One such strategy, the direct approach, results in a chirp family that is called the level-specific chirp." Data from studies using level-dependent chirps [6–11] are very encouraging, reporting ABRs recorded in less time and with higher amplitude values. The latter is very important for the statistical algorithms of the AABR devices, meaning that higher statistical accuracy can be obtained in the chirp-evoked AABRs.

3. Middle ear reflectance and Middle Ear Power Analysis (MEPA)

Data from studies that have evaluated the performance of NHS programs in the well-baby clinic or in the NICU [4, 12, 13] have reported that the majority of "screening refers" are due to transmission impeding factors such as the amniotic fluid or any substance blocking the propagation of the acoustic stimulus. Usually, these conditions are transient (i.e., they last 24–30 h), and infants can pass the OAE test when the fluid is absorbed or when the auditory meatus is clean.

Using a middle ear power analysis (MEPA) testing procedure, it is possible to determine whether the middle ear conducts properly acoustic stimuli, and in this context, the OAE screening results can be interpreted more clearly. Data from the literature [14, 15] have shown that one of the MEPA metrics, the middle ear reflectance, is more sensitive to the distortion product OAE (DPOAE) status than the 1-kHz tympanometry values. Power reflectance is a measure of middle ear inefficiency. It is the ratio or percentage of power reflected from the eardrum to the incident power as a function of frequency. Acoustic power measurements objectively quantify middle ear function or malfunction.

Currently, there is only one manufacturer (Mimosa Acoustics) offering reflectance measurements. The company offers two devices capable of MEPA, DPOAE, and general OAE measurements: the Otostat (handheld) and the HearID (research oriented) model. These devices (depicted in Figure 1) can measure wideband power reflectance up to 6 kHz and most importantly without the need for a pressurized ear canal.

To interpret the clinical usefulness of the MEPA approach, Hunter et al. [15] constructed normative regions for newborns, relating middle ear reflectance values evoked by chirp stimuli and DPOAE amplitudes at 1.0, 1.5, 2.0, 3.0, 4.0, and 6.0 kHz. The three regions were described as follows:

1. A retest area (where the values of reflectance are high)
2. An ambiguous area (where the values of reflectance are moderate)
3. A pass area (where the values of reflectance are low)

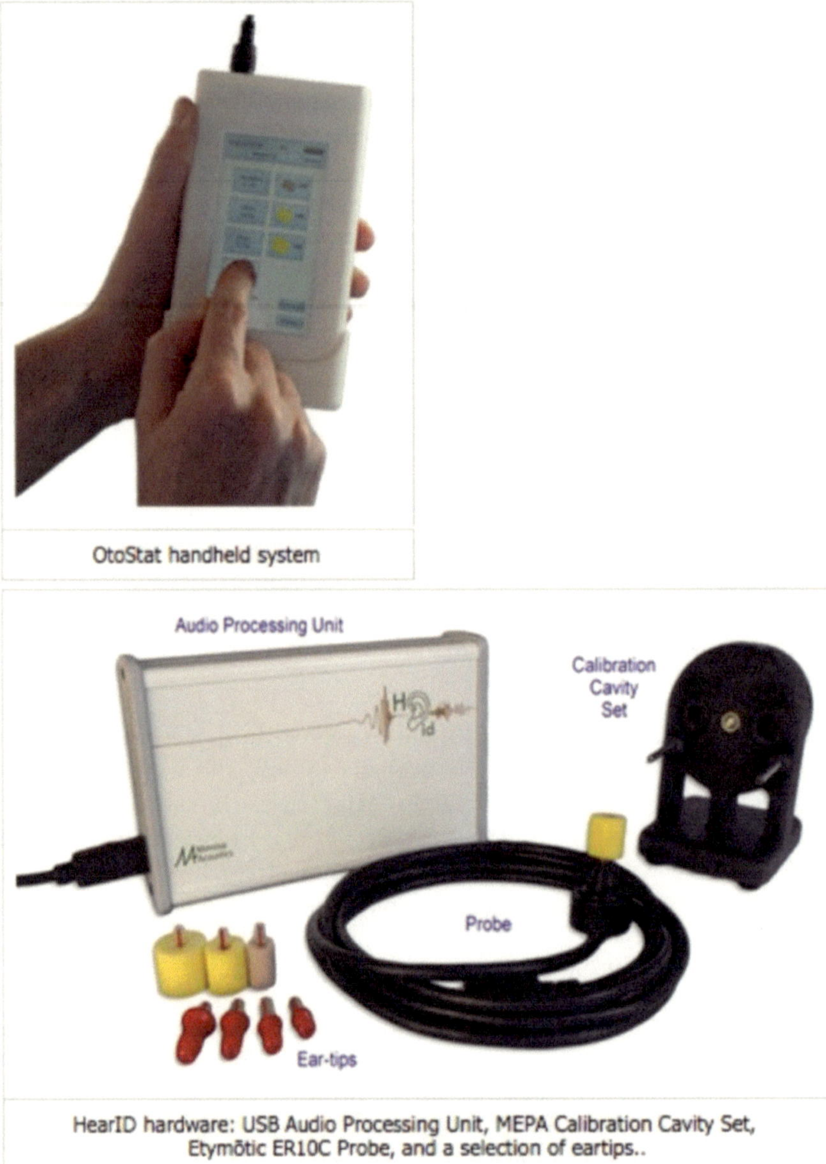

Figure 1. The Mimosa Acoustic devices capable of recording wideband reflectance and OAEs. Data from the Mimosa Acoustics website (http://www.mimosaacoustics.com).

These areas are depicted in Figure 2. In terms of interpretation, If the MEPA reflectance values fall above the "pass" area, especially around 2 kHz, outer or middle ear problems may be the cause, and a rescreening session after a few hours or a day is recommended prior to diagnostic referral. If the outcome is still a "refer" then clinical assessment is necessary. If the MEPA reflectance values fall within the "pass" area, especially around 2 kHz, the middle ear is more likely to be normal and associated with a DPOAE pass result. If the DPOAE result is ambiguous or a "refer", then middle ear issues are not suspected as a hearing deficit cause and further clinical assessment is necessary. Table 1 summarizes all these outcomes.

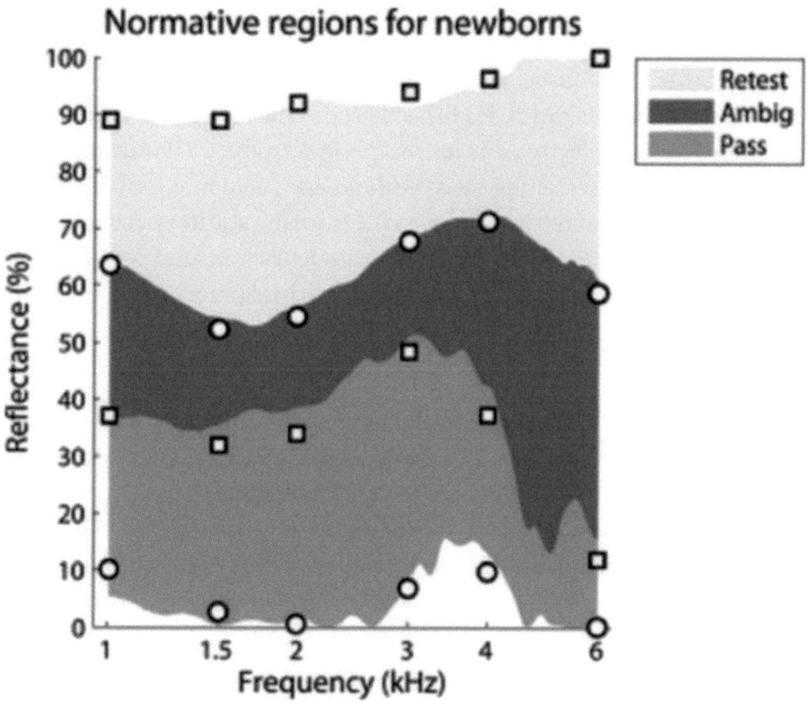

Figure 2. Pass, ambiguous, and retest regions for wideband reflectance using chirp (solid regions) and sine (symbols) stimuli. Results above this region, especially at 2 kHz, are associated with false-positive DPOAE refer results. Data from the Mimosa Acoustics website and from Hunter et al. (2010).

Overall DPOAE result	Reflectance at 2.0 kHz	Interpretation
Pass	In the pass area	Pass—normal result
Pass	Above the pass area (i.e., in the ambiguous or retest area)	Pass—may have middle ear issues, cochlear response normal
Refer	In the pass area	Refer—consistent with SNHL, requires follow-up
Refer	Above the pass area (i.e., in the ambiguous or retest areas)	Rescreening is suggested; repeat MEPA to determine status of the middle ear

Table 1. How to interpet distortion product OAEs and reflectance results in newborns (from http://www.mimosaacoustics.com).

4. Auditory Steady-State Responses (ASSR)

OAE and ABR testing procedures are evoked by electrical transient stimuli (clicks, filtered clicks, etc.), and as a result, the responses are correlated with a few audiometric frequencies, which correspond to the maximum spectral content of the stimulus (around 2.0 kHz). Considering this clinical setup, there are other protocols that could be candidates for a hearing assessment of neonates, children, and adults. Among those is the electrocochleography (EcoG), the middle latency (ML) responses, and the most recently reported steady-state responses (SSR). The first two approaches can be excluded because they require long times either for the position of an intratympanic electrode or for sampling purposes. The last protocol has shown a good potential for hearing screening since with an adequate manipulation of the stimulus modulation frequency, one can record responses or from the auditory cortex (low modulation frequencies around 40 Hz) or from the brainstem (frequencies around 50–120 Hz) [16–18]. The basic SSR protocol has evolved into an automated procedure (ASSR) where multiple stimulus frequencies are used and regression models predict hearing levels at the tested stimuli. The ASSR protocols have been greatly optimized for lower frequency stimuli such as 500 Hz [19].

In 2002, Conne-Wesson et al. [16] suggested that it could be possible to use an SSR protocol in a Neonatal Hearing Program, and since the SSR responses were generated by the brainstem for modulation frequencies >40 Hz, the ASSR could substitute the AABR [20–22]. In the referenced studies, a good agreement has been reported between the ASSR and the AABR responses at 2.0 kHz and various significant differences at 0.5, 1.0, and 4.0 kHz. The available data suggest that the AASR protocols should be developed further to become more independent of various clinical factors (related to the tested subject and to the stimuli used) and should be applied on a large population of subjects so that the results can be easily used clinically.

The important factors affecting the AABR responses (i.e., the ambient noise and the skin-electrode impedance) interfere also with the ASSR recordings. In 2010, Vivosonic presented a new family of devices (called amplitrodes) using a novel approach. Each scalp electrode was connected to a small preamplifier within the electrode assembly. Amplifying the signal in situ has many advantages, such as the suppression of the ambient noise and the elevation of the signal-to-noise ratio (S/N). This approach results in clean AABR and ASSR traces. One of the issues reported since its release, is that the new electrodes require very often a change of the electrode batteries.

In the context of a neonatal screening, an ASSR screening protocol can focus on discrete frequency points (i.e., 1.0 and 2.0 kHz or 2.0 and 4.0 kHz), which show relative immunity to ambient noise, as shown in the neonatal data in Figures 3A and 3B. One of the problems of the early ASSR devices (Audera by Viasys; Master by Natus) was that the mean hearing threshold estimates were characterized by large variance. Recent data in the literature and specifically from the Audix equipment developers (Neuronic) report significant advances both in terms of software and hardware and a superior performance of a multiple SSR protocol to the conventional ABR [23, 24].

http://dx.doi.org/10.5772/61178

A

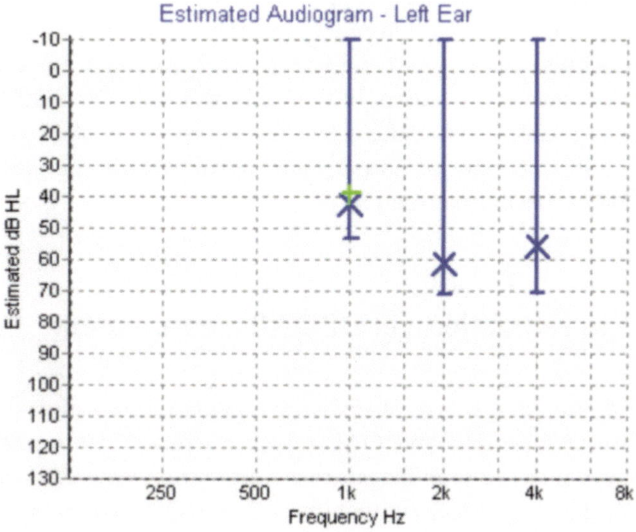

B

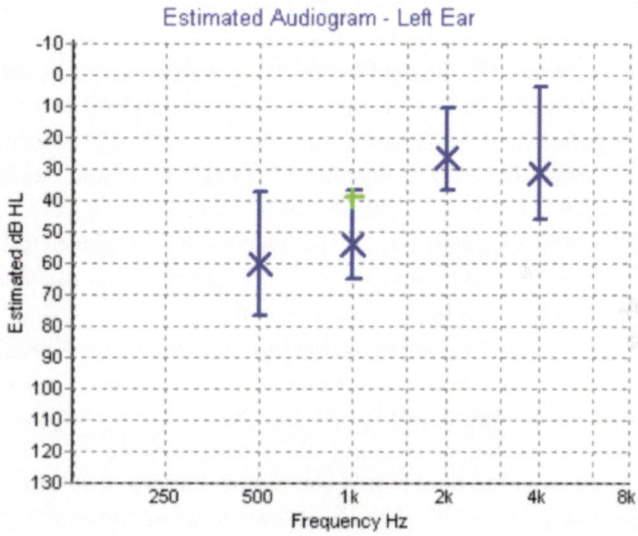

Figure 3. A) ASSR responses from a non-cooperative infant, using the AUDERA ASSR device (VIASYS). Responses at 500 Hz were not available due to noise caused by myogenic artifacts. The ASSR recording time was 14 min longer that the AABR test, resulting as 22 min. The large size of the error bars, at 2.0 and 4 kHz, show threshold means at 60 and 55 dB HL, but the variability of the measurements makes the threshold prediction difficult to be considered. (B) ASSR response from another well-baby infant, using the same ASSR device. The ASSR recording was also significantly longer than the AABR response (16 vs. 7 min). The error bars around the threshold average (indicated by an "x") are small and the prediction can be considered practical. For example, at 1.0 kHz, the threshold level is shown at 55 dB with a 95% probability that it will be in the interval 35–65 dB HL. The latter estimates are derived from the values of the error bars.

Recently, a study by Ciorba et al. [25] presented data on the relationship between ABR, ASSR estimates, and data from Conditioned Orientation Responses (COR), a technique widely diffused in the intervention phase of many UNHS programs. The data suggested a very good relationship between the outcomes of the ASSR and the COR techniques, with the ASSR data being closer to the ABR estimates. Data from large-scale studies along this direction (i.e., comparing ASSR with other protocols) could support this hypothesis and eliminate the use of ABR and COR in this intervention step.

5. Threshold estimation via DPOAE measurements

From the early nineties, where OAEs were accepted in the clinical practice, the relationship between hearing threshold and OAE responses received a lot of attention [26–28]. What previous research suggests is that in cases presenting sensorineural deficits (i.e., excluding conductive and retrocochlear causes), there is a good agreement between the OAE respond levels and the hearing threshold. In this context, distortion product OAE (DPOAE) protocols can provide additional information [26, 29–31]. Input–output (or I/O functions) DPOAE protocols provide information on the relationship between the evoking stimulus and the signal compression of the cochlear amplifier. Data supporting this hypothesis are derived from animal experiments (furosemide intoxication) [32] and clinical human studies from cases presenting sensorineural deficits [29, 33–34]. When the hearing loss is increased, the slope of the corresponding DPOAE I/O-functions decreases and reveals a loss of compression in the cochlear amplifier. Using various setups of the DPOAE I/O stimuli, one can estimate the cochlear compression, which is related to a specific threshold value [31, 35]. Janssen et al. [36] used this concept to produce a relationship between DPOAE I/O amplitude values and hearing threshold. According to their data, "The hearing threshold was found to be increasing within the early postnatal period (average age: 3 days), predominantly at the higher frequencies, and to be normalized in a follow-up measurement (after four weeks). However, the slope of the DPOAE I/O-functions obtained in the first and second measurement was unchanged revealing normal cochlear compression. Consequently, these findings were interpreted as temporary conductive hearing losses due to the presence of amniotic fluid and/or Eustachian tube dysfunction." The value of cochlear compression changes when the middle ear stimulus pathway is affected. Therefore, this procedure has the theoretical potential to discriminate middle from inner ear deficits. Data from the literature have not validated yet this hypothesis.

The research findings from Janssen et al. [36] and Gorga et al. [35] have been commercialized by Natus in the Cochlea-Scan device [37]. Hearing threshold can be extrapolated up to values relative to 50 dB HL in the frequency range from 1.5 to 6 kHz. Figure 4 shows a typical hearing threshold profile and the corresponding Cochlea-Scan-mediated estimation of hearing threshold. At present, the Cochlea-Scan device offers a platform for a third-generation OAE testing (TEOAEs and DPOAEs), I/O DPOAE estimation with hearing threshold extrapolation.

Further analyses [38, 39] on the efficacy of the Cochlea-Scan DPOAE algorithm, relating hearing threshold data and Cochlea-Scan estimated thresholds from a group of adult sensor-

http://dx.doi.org/10.5772/61178

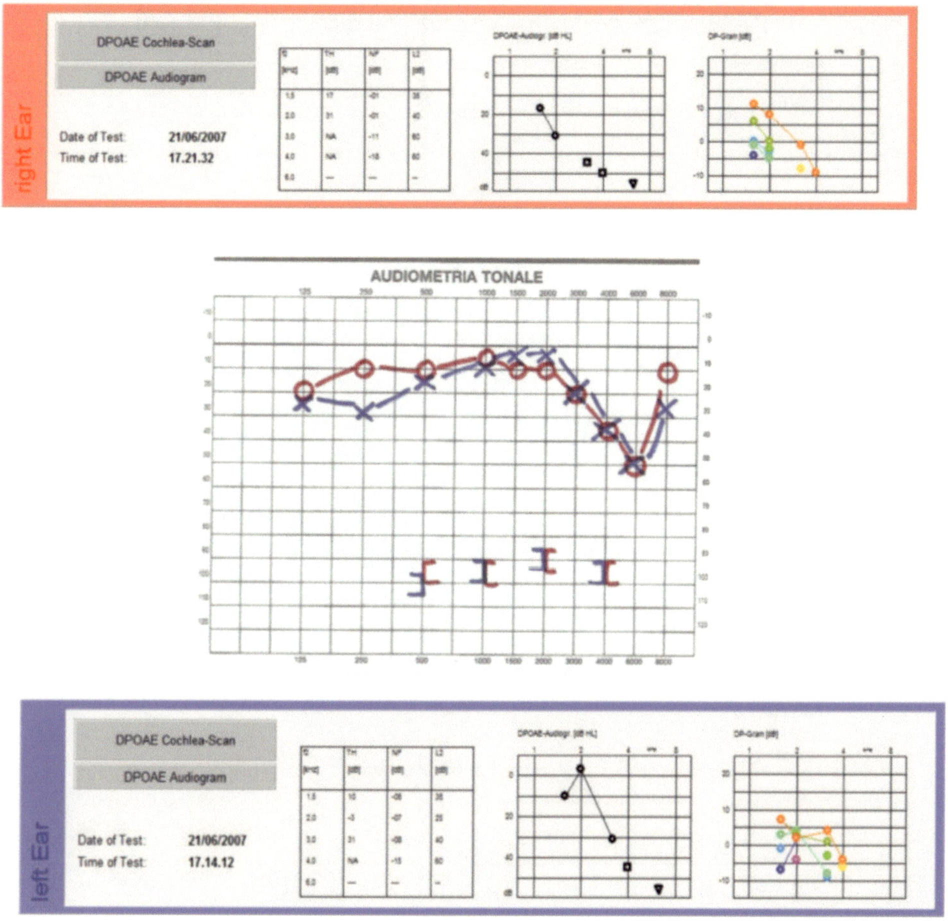

Figure 4. Cochlea-Scan data in comparison to behavioral threshold levels, from an adult subject. Top panel: Cochlea-Scan responses and threshold estimation from the right ear; middle panel: behavioral data; bottom panel: Cochlea-Scan responses and threshold estimation from the left ear. The Cochlea-Scan panels report the estimated threshold values per frequency. The acronym "NA" means that at the specific frequency no threshold estimation was possible.

ineural cases, suggested a different scenario than the one proposed initially by Janssen et al. [36]. In the Hatzopoulos et al. [39] study, behavioral and Cochlea-Scan data were analyzed with logistic regression models in order to find the probability (≤0.9) of a robust DPOAE response at 2.0, 3.0, and 4.0 kHz. The data suggested that the maximum behavioral levels where valid DPOAEs could be detected were equal to of 32.8, 21, and 34 dB, respectively. For normal hearing adults, the detection levels were lower. Figures 5 and 6 depict the relationship between behavioral data (at 2.0, 3.0, and 4.0 kHz) and Cochlea-Scan estimates from the cases presenting hearing loss. For example, in Figure 5 and for 2.0 kHz, a probability of 90% Cochlea-Scan response detection corresponds to a threshold approximately of 15 dB HL. In this context, it is still possible to have a detection threshold as high as 50 dB HL. The corresponding probability falls below 30% and, as such, limits the usefulness of the Cochlea-Scan protocol

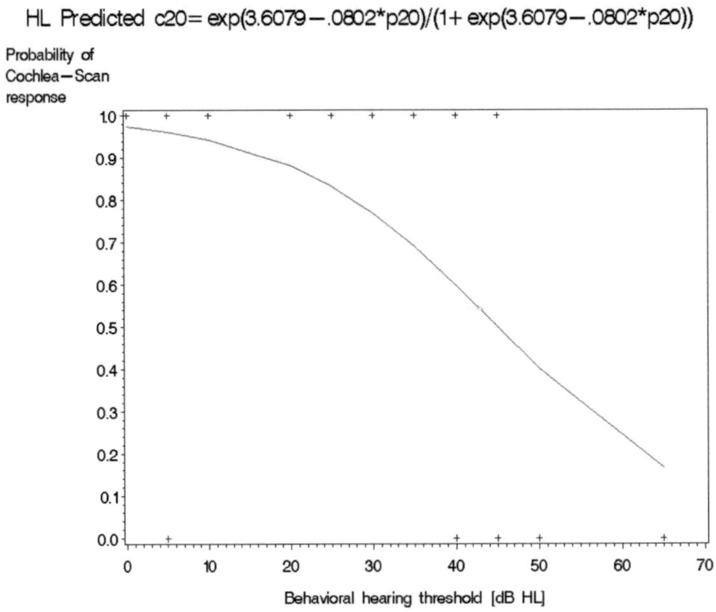

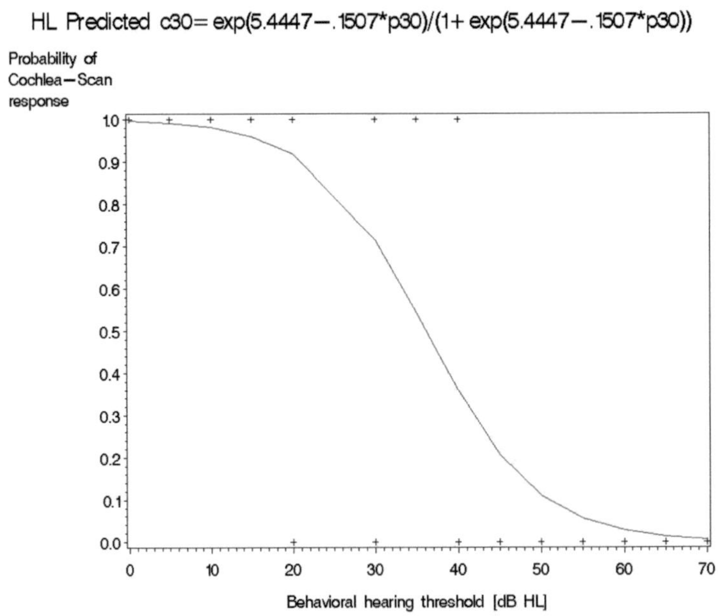

Figure 5. Logistic regression model for normal hearing threshold Cochlea-Scan data at 2.0 and 3.0 kHz. The equation relating the two variables (c = Cochlea-Scan; p = behavioral threshold) is shown at the top of each graph. The x axis shows behavioral threshold in dB HL and the y axis the probability of a Cochlea-Scan response. For a fixed response probability of 90%, the detectable threshold level is approximately 15 and 20 dB HL, for the data at 2.0 and 3.0 kHz. This implies that in order to obtain a Cochlea-Scan response for a 50-dB HL hearing threshold, the probability of finding a true response drops to 40% and 10%, respectively (for 2.0 and 3.0 kHz).

http://dx.doi.org/10.5772/61178

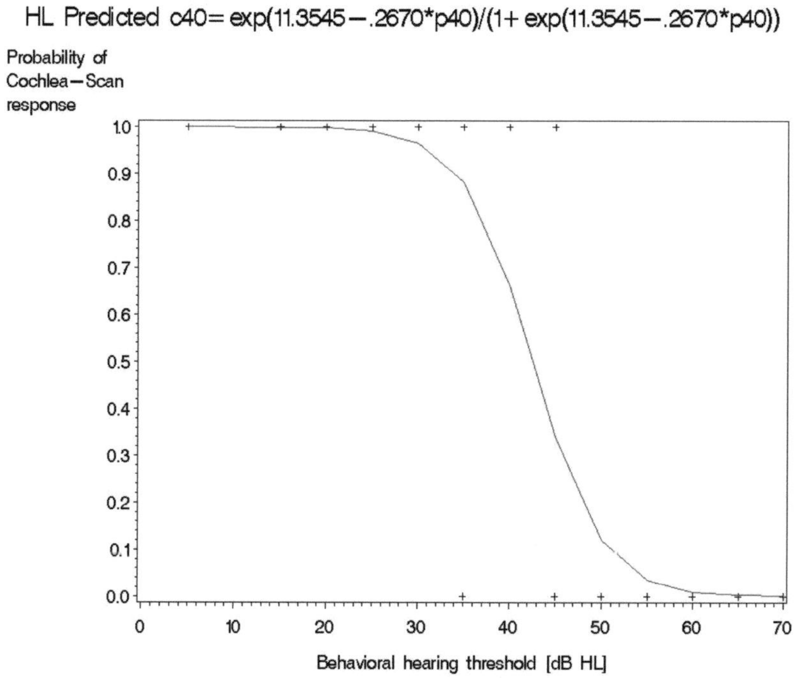

Figure 6. Logistic regression model for normal hearing threshold Cochlea-Scan data at 4.0 kHz. The equation relating the two variables (c = Cochlea-Scan; p = behavioral threshold) is shown at the top of each graph. The x axis shows behavioral threshold in dB HL and the y axis the probability of a Cochlea-Scan response. For a fixed response probability of 90%, the detectable threshold level is approximately 35 dB HL. For a 50-dB HL threshold, the probability of a true response drops to 15%. The relationship between the behavioral and the Cochlea-Scan data at 4.0 kHz is optimized, but the sensitivity of the method drops very quickly as we move to higher thresholds 35 dB HL.

The authors at this point in time could not verify if Natus has intentions of developing further this product. Cochlea-Scan threshold estimation could be greatly improved by introducing changes in the device's algorithms related to (i) the sample size, which was used to calibrate the prototype device. Sampling a larger population can minimize the variance of the average DPOAE amplitude per tested frequency (ii) by inserting correction factors in the algorithm, which extrapolates DPOAE amplitudes to hearing levels. Janssen et al. [36] have used a linear regression model to achieve this, but higher-order models (quadratic, cubic) can offer higher precision in the threshold estimation.

6. Integration of multiple hearing assessment protocols into an automated device

The success of the NHS screening practices challenged another area of pediatric audiology, the area of schoolchildren screening. Data from large-scale screening programs, as in Poland, suggested that in this area different protocols could be applied than in UNHS programs, with emphasis on pure tone behavioral responses, tympanometry, and ABR [40]. The OAEs were found the less effective tool in the battery of screening tests, suffering mainly from the ambient noise present in schools.

Recently, the fifth-generation OAE equipment appeared in the market. A number of OAE manufacturers (Natus, Path Medical solutions) proposed handheld devices capable of testing subjects with OAEs/AOAEs, AABR, and ASSR. A tympanometry assessment has not appeared so far due to complications in the probe of the device (canal pressurization issues). Mimosa Acoustics offers wide-reflectance measurements (which can substitute acoustic immittance) and OAEs but not evoked potentials.

The proposal from Path Medical Solutions (model: Sentiero—advanced) is a device capable not only of AOAE/AABR/ASSR protocols but also of protocols for speech Audiometry. The device is depicted in Figure 7. Such a device can be easily implemented in both phases (identification and intervention) of a UNHS program, and it is hoped that other manufacturers will follow this protocol-integration trend.

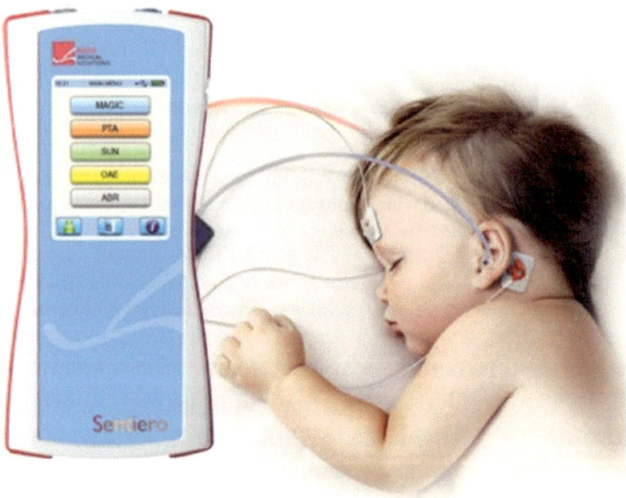

Figure 7. The Sentiero Advanced device (data from the website of Path medical solutions http://www.pathme.de).

7. Conclusions

During the last 10–15 years, significant advances have been made toward the integration of various protocols and technologies in UNHS strategies. The most important contribution is in the area of auditory steady-state responses, which has been shown to be well correlated with other metrics in audiology such as the AABR, ABR, OAEs, and COR. The current technological trends call for an integration of even more protocols and algorithms in a handheld device. The clinical robustness and response quality of these new entries is yet to be evaluated.

http://dx.doi.org/10.5772/61178

8. Appendix

The reader interested in additional information than the one presented might visit the OAE Portal (http://www.otoemissions.org) and the OAE Portal Forum.

Author details

Stavros Hatzopoulos[1], Henryk Skarzynski[2] and Piotr H Skarzynski[2,3,4]

1 Department of Audiology and ENT, University of Ferrara, Italy

2 Institute of Physiology and Pathology of Hearing, Warsaw, Poland

3 Heart Failure and Cardiac Rehabilitation Department of the Medical University of Warsaw, Poland

4 Institute of Sensory Organs, Kajetany, Poland

References

[1] Kemp DT. Stimulated acoustic emissions from within the human auditory system. J Acoust Soc Am. 1978:1386–91.

[2] Robinette M and Glattke T editors. Otoacoustic Emissions: Clinical Applications. New York: Thieme; 1997.

[3] Ciorba A, Hatzopoulos S, Camurri L, Negossi L, Rossi M, Cosso D, and Martini A. Neonatal newborn hearing screening: four years of experience at the Ferrara University Hospital (cheap project). Acta Otorhinolaryngol Ital, 2007;27:10–16.

[4] White KR, Vohr BR, Meyer S, Widen JE, Johnson JL, Gravel JS, James M, Kennalley T, Maxon AB, Spivak L, Sullivan-Mahoney M, Weirather Y. A multisite study to examine the efficacy of the otoacoustic emission/automated auditory brainstem response newborn hearing screening protocol: research design and results of the study. Am J Audiol. 2005;14:186–199.

[5] Kristensen SG, Elberling C. Auditory brainstem responses to level-specific chirps in normal-hearing adults. J Am Acad Audiol 2012; 23:712–721.

[6] Ferm I, Lighfoot G, Stevens J. Comparison of ABR response amplitude, test time and estimation of hearing threshold using specific chirp and tone pip stimuli in newborns. Int J Audiol 2013;52:419–423.

[7] Rodriguez GR, Ramos N, Lewis DR. Comparing auditory brainstem responses to toneburst and narrow band CE-chirp in young infants. Int J Pediatr Otorhinolaryngol 2013;77:1555–1560.

[8] Zirn S, Louza J, Reiman V, Wittlinger N, Hempel JM, Schuster M. Comparison between ABR with click and narrow band chirp stimuli in children. Int J Pediatr Otorhinolaryngol 2014; 78:1352–1355.

[9] Cebulla M, Lurz H, Shehata-Dieler W. Evaluation of waveform, latency and amplitude values of chirp ABR in newborns. Int J Pediatr Otorhinolaryngol 2014; 78: 762–768.

[10] Rodriguez GR, Lewis DR. Establishing auditory steady-state response thresholds to narrow band CE-chirps in full term neonates. Int J Pediatr Ororhinolaryngol 2014;78:238–243.

[11] Stuart A, Cobb KM. Effect of stimulus and number of sweeps on the neonate auditory brainstem response. Ear Hear 2014;35:585–588.

[12] Aithal S, Aithal V, Kei J, Driscoll C. Conductive hearing loss and middle ear pathology in young infants referred through a newborn universal hearing screening program in Australia. J Am Acad Audiol 2012 23: 673–685.

[13] Vos B, Lagasse R, Leveque A. Main outcomes of a newborn hearing screening program in Belgium over six years. Int J Pediatr Otorhinolaryngol 2014 78:1496–1502.

[14] Sanford C, Keefe D, Liu YW, Fitzpatrick D, McCreery R, Lewis D, and Gorga M. Sound-conduction effects on distortion-product otoacoustic emission screening outcomes in newborn infants: test performance of wideband acoustic transfer functions and 1 kHz tympanometry. Ear Hear 2009;30: 635–652.

[15] Hunter L, Feeney P, Miller JL, Jeng P, and Bohning S. Wideband reflectance in newborns. Normative regions and relationship to hearing-screening results. Ear Hear 2010;31:599–610.

[16] Cone-Wesson B, Dowell R, Tomlin D, Rance G, Ming Wu. The auditory steady state response. Comparisons with the auditory brainstem response. J Am Acad Audiol 2002; 13: 173–187.

[17] Dimitrijevic A, John S, Roon P, et al. Estimating the audiogram using multiple auditory steady state responses. J Am Acad Audiol 2002; 13: 205–224.

[18] John MS, Picton TW. Human auditory steady-state responses to amplitude-modulated tones: phase and latency measurements. Hear Res 2000; 141: 57–79.

[19] Gorga MP, Neely ST, Hoover BM, Dierking DM, Beauchaine KL, Manning C. Determining the upper limits of stimulation for auditory steady-state response measurements. Ear Hear. 2004;25:302–307.

[20] Stueve MP, O'Rourke C. Estimation of hearing loss in children: comparison of auditory steady-state response, auditory brainstem response, and behavioral test methods. Am J Audiol. 2003;12:125–136.

[21] Luts H, Desloovere C, Kumar A, Vandermeersch E, Wouters J. Objective assessment of frequency-specific hearing thresholds in babies. Int J Pediatr Otorhinolaryngol. 2004 68(7):915–926.

[22] Swanepoel D, Hugo R, Roode R. Auditory steady-state responses for children with severe to profound hearing loss. Arch Otolaryngol Head Neck Surg. 2004;130:531–535.

[23] MIjares E, Perez Abalo MC, Herrera D, Lage A, Vega M. Comparing statistics for objective detection of transient and steady-state evoked responses in newborns. Int J Audiol 2013;52:44–49.

[24] Perez Abalo MC, Rogriguez E, Sanchez M, Santos E, Torres Fortuny A. New system for neonatal hearing screening based on auditory steady state responses. J Med Eng Technol 2013;37:368 374.

[25] Ciorba A, Hatzopoulos S, Petruccelli J, Mazzoli M, Pastore A, Kochanek K, Skarzynski P, Wlodarczyk A and Skarzynski H.Identifying congenital hearing impairment: preliminary results from a comparative study using objective and subjective audiometric protocols. Acta Otorhinolaryngol Ital 2013;33:29–35.

[26] Whitehead ML, McCoy MJ, Lonsbury-Martin BL, Martin GK. Dependence of distortion-product otoacoustic emissions in primary tone level in normal and impaired ears. I. Effects of decreasing L2 below L1. J Acoust Soc Am 1995a 97: 2346–2358.

[27] Whitehead ML, Stagner BB, Lonsbury-Martin BL, Martin GK. Effects of ear-canal standing waves on measurements of distortion-product otoacoustic emissions. J Acoust Soc Am 1995b 98: 3202–3214

[28] Shera CA, Guinan JJ Jr. Evoked otoacoustic emissions arise by two fundamentally different mechanisms: a taxonomy for mammalian OAEs. J Acoust Soc Am. 1999;105:782–798.

[29] Janssen T, Kummer P, Arnold W. Growth behavior of the 2f1-f2 distortion product otoacoustic emission in tinnitus. J Acoust Soc Am 1998;103 (6):3418–3430.

[30] Dorn PA, Konrad-Martin D, Neely ST, Keefe DH, Cyr E, Gorga MP. Distortion product otoacoustic emission input/output functions in normal-hearing and hearing-impaired human ears. J Acoust Soc Am. 2001;110:3119–3131.

[31] Gorga MP, Neely ST, Dierking DM, Dorn PA, Hoover BM, Fitzpatrick DF. Distortion product otoacoustic emission suppression tuning curves in normal-hearing and hearing-impaired human ears. J Acoust Soc Am. 2003b;114(1):263–278.

[32] Mills DM, Rubel ED. Development of the cochlear amplifier. J Acoust Soc Am 1996; 100: 428–441.

[33] Kummer P, Janssen T, Arnold W. The level and growth behavior of the 2f1-f2 distortion product otoacoustic emission and its relationship to auditory sensitivity in normal hearing and cochlear hearing loss. J Acoust Soc Am 1998;103 (6):3431–3444.

[34] Boege P, Janssen T. Pure-tone threshold estimation from extrapolated distortion product otoacoustic emission I/O-functions in normal and cochlear hearing loss ears. J Acoust Soc Am 2002 111: 1810–1818.

[35] Gorga MP, Neely ST, Dorn PA, Hoover BM. Further efforts to predict pure-tone thresholds from distortion product otoacoustic emission input/output functions. J Acoust Soc Am 2003a;113:3275–3284.

[36] Janssen T, Klein A, Gehr D. Automatische Hörschwellenbestimung bei Neugeborenen mit extrapolierten DPOAE-Wachstumsfunktionen. Eine neue Hörscreening-Methode. HNO 2003 16 : 125-128

[37] Oswald JA, Janssen T Weighted DPOAE I/O-functions: a tool for automatically assessing hearing loss in clinical application. Z Med Physik 2003; 13: 93–98.

[38] Hatzopoulos S, Petruccelli J, Ciorba A and Martini A. Optimizing otoacoustic emission protocols for a UNHS program. Audiol Neurotol 2009;14(1):7–16.

[39] Hatzopoulos S, Ciorba A, Petruccelli J, Grasso D, Sliwa L, Skarzynski H and Martini A. Estimation of the Hearing Threshold Using behavioral Audiometry, CochleaScan and ASSR protocols Int J Audiol 2009;48:625–631.

[40] Sliwa L, Hatzopoulos S, Kochanek K, Piłka A, SenderskiA and Henryk Skarzynski. A comparison of audiometric and objective methods in hearing screening of school children. A preliminary study. Int J Pediatr Otorhinolaryngol 2011;75: 483–488.

Section 6

Hearing Loss and Cochlear Implants

Chapter 10

Bilateral Cochlear Implants, Minimizing Auditory Rehabilitation

Miguel A. Hyppolito and Eduardo T. Massuda

Additional information is available at the end of the chapter

http://dx.doi.org/10.5772/61228

Abstract

Bilateral cochlear implant has increased in recent years due to benefits such as the location of the sign, decrease in head shadow effect, and binaural summation. The aim of this chapter is to discuss issues related to the bilateral cochlear implant costs and benefits and its reflections on auditory rehabilitation, allowing the reader to do a search and strengthen it scientifically with this issue, giving theoretical foundation to better guide and advise their patients.

Keywords: Bilateral cochlear implants, rehabilitation, social impact, individual impact, hearing aids

1. Introduction

Hearing loss has an important impact on people's lives, especially in cases of severe and profound hearing loss. In developed countries, approximately one to two children per 1,000 have moderate to profound bilateral sensorineural hearing loss. Sensorineural hearing loss can be classified as hereditary, acquired, or idiopathic, and acquired environmental etiology is present in approximately 35% [1].

Hearing is an important key to the oral language acquisition and to the world perception. Children who are not exposed to language stimulation in the first years of life will present a lag in their auditory and linguistic development. The first years of life are critical for the greatest neuronal plasticity in the auditory pathway as it is the period of the development of auditory and language skills. Depending on the auditory external stimulus, the central auditory nervous system can be changed positively or negatively. In addition, the period of receipt of hearing linguistic symbols is a prerequisite to form the oral communication [2].

Hearing loss restrict the entry of sounds that will change the auditory development and consequently the language.

In most cases of sensorineural hearing loss, the first site of lesion is inside the cochlea, with results in insufficient energy transduction of the acoustic mechanism of neural impulses to the auditory nerve. In some cases, conventional hearing aids are not enough to restore the hearing; cochlear implant could be indicated.

2. The role of bilateral cochlear implant and rehabilitation process

The cochlear implant is considered the only high-tech device capable of converting acoustic signals into electrical stimuli, causing auditory sensation through direct stimulation of the auditory nerve. It is considered the most effective sensory prosthesis in the history of medicine (Figure 1).

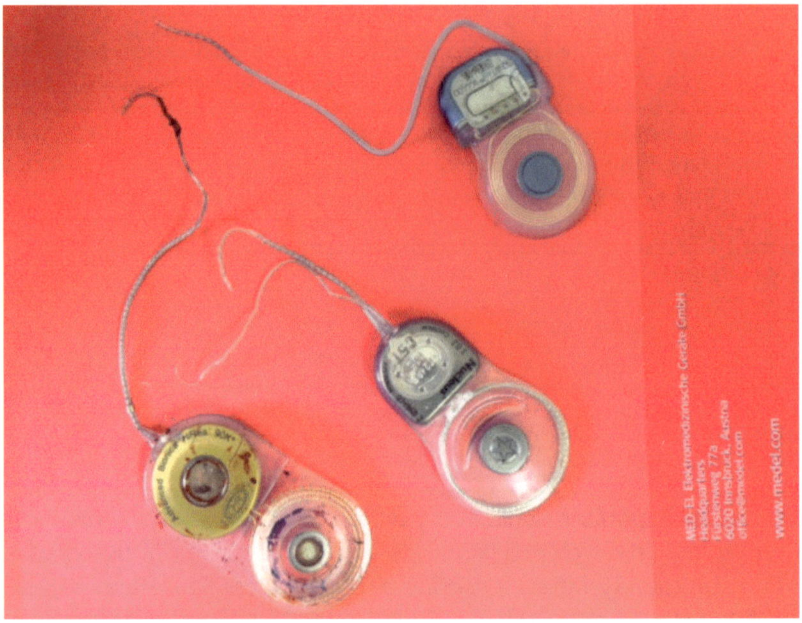

Figure 1. The cochlear implant system. Internal device implant of various manufacturers.

Cochlear implant results allow listening sensation and access to oral language. Its users can do speech acquisition and development of auditory and language skills. In humans, variability in the results is evident. An important detail and worthy of emphasis is the fact that the earlier the intervention occurs, the better the result reached with the use of the cochlear implant [3].

In the USA, cochlear implants were approved for adults with postlingual (hearing loss after 4 years old) severe to profound hearing loss in 1985 [4], and 10 years later, it was approved for adults with prelingual deafness (hearing loss before 4 years old) [5].

Developments in the indication criteria suffer direct interference of the constant technological development along with the improvement of surgical techniques and training and qualification of interdisciplinary teams.

Children who receive the cochlear implant early, until 2 years old, often present an appropriate oral language development, which is similar to the child who does not present any deficiency in the hearing [6, 7].

Based on the current knowledge on patients who received unilateral cochlear implants with good results, which provide normal hearing to the implanted ear, the majority of these patients have some difficulties on sound location and sound discrimination abilities in noisy environments. When evaluated by the hearing in noise test (HINT), patients are required to use both ears together (binaural hearing) to repeat sentences. Unilateral cochlear implant users have greater effort to conversation in noise because binaural hearing ability is essential for communication in noisy settings and for other aspects of functional hearing, such as sound localization and recognition of environmental sounds [8].

The benefits of the unilateral cochlear implants are evidenced by several studies in the literature [9-13].

Studies have shown that children with bilateral cochlear implants have better sensitivity for the perception of sounds and improvement in the quality of speech [14-16].

Studies comparing the use of bilateral cochlear implants with unilateral cochlear implants associated with a hearing aid in the other ear on children had shown that the bilateral cochlear implant brings better educational benefits in terms of academic results. Children who were implanted before attending the school have a greater propensity to achieve better academic results and be in regular education than those deployed after reaching school age [15-17].

The studies in the systematic review present that the procedure of bilateral implantation is relatively recent and that little research on these results is available [18]. The existing studies on bilateral cochlear implant have approached diversified topics, such as language, communication, and quality-of-life measures. Important results pointed out the benefit of bilateral implantation in children, among them, father-and-son interaction and school performance [19-22].

The additional benefits provided by the second implant considering costs and additional risks, such as additional hardware expense, surgical risk, and programming time, need to be considered [23].

A study that examined the cost utility of postlingual children and adults concluded that quality of life is likely to be obtained per unit of expenditure deployment with unilateral than bilateral implantation [24].

For adults, there was no significant change in quality of life with the second CI than with the first CI. However, these results cannot be extrapolated to children due to the very different nature of auditory stimulation for prelingually deaf children when we consider the neuroplasticity of the central nervous system and synaptic neuronal remodeling with the binaural auditory stimulation, which will become important for speech acquisition and language development around 5 years old, like normal hearing children reflecting on learning, especially in the school environment. These studies could be important in determining the benefits of the second implant to children in school, in the family, and in social environments.

With a unilateral cochlear implant, individuals have some limitations in the ability to perceive multiple sound entries with segregated independent sources, and this situation reflects a difficulty in understanding speech in the presence of competitive signals (noise) and to the location of the sound in the environment. To improve this condition to understand difficulties in the presence of noise and localization of sound source, thousands of patients have sought the bilateral cochlear implant [25].

Several studies have demonstrated better performance resulting from the use of the bilateral cochlear implant to identify sounds within a multispeaker environment [26-28].

The magnitude and the type of advantage of the cochlear implant are not universal. Comparing the performance of unilateral versus bilateral hearing conditions with cochlear implants, head shadow effect, squelch effect, and binaural summation are three situations that contribute significantly to improve speech understanding, especially in environments with noise and sound location, because the central auditory pathways on the brainstem can differentiate sound characteristics in seconds, which arrive in each ear as an auditory reflex.

The following three hearing conditions must be defined:

1. Head shadow effect. This is defined as a physical phenomenon and head blocks the arrival of sound in the hearing ear from different locations, which allows the listener to hear using the ear with better signal-to-noise ratio (SNR).

2. Binaural redundancy or binaural summation. This is a result of the central auditory processing of the sound entries on both ears at the same time and is analyzed in the central auditory pathways of the brainstem. This reflects the ability of the auditory nervous system to integrate and use bilateral auditory information for better performance than in a single ear.

3. Squelch effect. This reflects the ability of the auditory brainstem to use bilateral auditory information when words or speech in noise sources are spatially separated using the ear with worse signal-to-noise ratio [29].

Bilateral cochlear implant users easily locate sounds, and they are also able to understand speech in noise. These individuals have a good performance of speech intelligibility and location, and binaural hearing is being used in such a way to facilitate their performance [30].

There is a critical period for the binaural auditory development for early simultaneous deployment when the evidences of plasticity of central auditory pathways act as soon as early bilateral implantation and differences are observed in the electrophysiological studies in children implanted bilaterally in sequence, even when the second implant was performed in a time interval shorter than 1 year [31, 32].

Children who received simultaneous bilateral cochlear implant between 5 and 18 months of age and used cochlear implant for 9 to 12 months achieved a result of auditory and language development equal to the listener children with the same chronological age. Therefore, children with prelingual deafness may develop oral expressive and receptive language within the normal range if they are implanted early [30].

In adults, both simultaneous and sequential bilateral cochlear implants improve comfort of listening with additional benefits besides the location of sound because two ears are getting auditory sensations [33].

For the best rehabilitation and greater opportunity for the development of speech and language, benefits minimizing the time of bilateral deafness are important, and the sequential cochlear implant in children will decrease as a result of the increase in the time interval between the first and the second contralateral implant. In this way, good benefits in word recognition and sound location begin in the first 12 months after cochlear implants and continue to occur over time [34].

Therefore, bilateral cochlear implant could be indicated to the following (Table 1):

- Children above 5 and 18 months of age with bilateral severe to profound sensorineural hearing loss less than 80 dB NA on the better ear, absence of cognitive impairment, and autism
- Individuals older than 5 years with severe to profound bilateral sensorineural postlingual hearing loss less than 80 dB NA on the better ear, with linguistic code established, first cochlear implant surgery performed up to 2 years of age, and interval between the first and the second implant not exceeding 5 years with no cognitive impairment and autism
- Individuals with severe to profound bilateral sensorineural postlingual hearing loss less than 80 dB NA on the better ear using cochlear implant in contralateral ear for at least 1 year, excepted in meningitis
- Individuals with severe to profound bilateral sensorineural hearing loss less than 80 dB NA in the better ear and blindness.

Age	Hearing loss level	Bilateral hearing losses	dB (better ear)	Cognitive impairment	Speech acquisition	CI intervals
5-18 months	Severe to profound	Present	<80	Negative	Prelingual	-
>5 years	Severe to profound	Present	<80	Negative	Postlingual	<5 years
>18 years	Severe to profound	Present	<80	Negative	Postlingual	>1 years
All ages	Severe to profound	Present	<80	Negative blindness*	Pre- or postlingual	-

* Two-sensory disability.

Table 1. Bilateral cochlear implant indications.

The best time and age for the CI surgery should be well discussed with the cochlear implant program team, which will have an early intervention for better hearing conditions in every way as its goal, providing individual hearing benefits and early social inclusion.

Some papers report that financial issues are not a problem to bilateral cochlear implant. Although it would benefit all children with deep bilateral sensorineural deafness, children will not be subject to additional risks with simultaneous CI. Moreover, if the benefit of the second implant is small, it is not worth the cost, and health systems and doctors will consider the cost-effectiveness issue [34]. The coverage by insurance providers is growing for bilateral implants.

Some points in the rehabilitation of individuals with bilateral cochlear implant should be considered in aiming to understand the speech and functional integration of each implant, resulting in a balanced binaural hearing that requires an effective hearing rehabilitation work. To all rehabilitation process, it is important to consider that each is an individual user and there are factors that affect the end result. Creating positive auditory experiences and selecting appropriate activities for every hearing age and skill are important to each individual. Adults, parents, and teachers should always have extra batteries available, and the speech therapist should show the importance of hearing practice through interactions of structured natural speech and hearing therapy.

The reeducational process involves relearning to listen, interpret, and process the sound information and speech. This way, the speech therapist should check separately each ear using the Ling Sounds or auditory discrimination until the user is able to identify when one of the implants is not working or when the batteries fail, establish specific goals for each ear separately or for binaural hearing based on speech acoustics and auditory development, check if parents or users understood the goals and reasons for this rehabilitation process, monitor all the progress and inform the user and the parents of the improvements in auditory skills and pay special attention to the practice to recommended individual therapy. The expectations in the following progress are the recognition in closed to open set, the recognition from predictable to unpredictable information, the recognition of familiar to unfamiliar words, the use of repetition to nonrepetition, the recognition of close to more distant sounds, and the recognition in quiet to noisy environments.

With the simultaneous CI implantation, users use two implants all the time. However, if a great discrepancy between the two ears is present, the worse ear is trained at a specific time.

To sequential CI implantation, the last ear implanted should get the maximum benefit from the bilateral cochlear implant to balance the second hearing competence with the first implant. The integration of the two ears is important to rehabilitation because together they contribute to daily hearing [14]. The rehabilitation process in the second implanted ear must be continued until the score of speech perception of the second implant is next to the first one or achieved good open set scores on speech recognition in a quiet environment. In some situations, the second implant will never reach the first [14].

For the guidance of the individual and his or her family as well as the rehabilitation in sequential CI, it is important that parents and users understand that the initial hearing perception of the implanted ear must be on the basic level and not on advanced skills as the first implant. Moreover, current research indicates that progress is faster with the second than the first implant, and both implants must be used every day in all environments and with news and complex information. The therapist must create some situations to demonstrate the benefit of two implants as in location, noise, or speech tests in different environments. If the child is under 3 years of age, it is recommended to use both implants all the time. If no perception or auditory discrimination is observed, hearing practice training with the newer implant or with the worst result implant is recommended.

Cochlear implant studies have shown that the bilateral cochlear implant indicated at an early age in children with profound bilateral prelingual deafness, considering the clinical conditions, etiologies, and surgical conditions of the deployment, has important benefits in overcoming and legitimating the costs and expenses of children under the same rehabilitation process. It is expected that these children acquire the same skills as 5-year-old children without deafness. The early bilateral cochlear implantation is important to the central auditory system plasticity response to the new electrical stimulation. The input of new auditory information on both ears is important in understanding speech and specific environmental situations like music, and several studies have shown the benefits of "head shadow effect" and binaural summation on bilateral cochlear implant users. Bilateral cochlear implanted individuals have better speech recognition in noise and sound localization with bilateral cochlear implant compared to a single implant. The roles of the multidisciplinary team in minimizing risks and optimizing the benefits of bilateral cochlear implant are important to be involved in indication and rehabilitation for better speech results with no significant risks. Therefore, bilaterally implanted patients generally report greater satisfaction with their bilateral implants compared with the unilateral situation. They describe better clarity, greater ease of listening, and better hearing overall.

Acknowledgements

We wish to thank the HCRP-FMRP-USP (FAEPA) for their support in teaching, research, and assistance.

Author details

Miguel A. Hyppolito* and Eduardo T. Massuda

*Address all correspondence to: mahyppo@fmrp.usp.br

Department of Otorhinolaryngology, Ophthalmology and Head and Neck Surgery, Ribeirão Preto Medical School, University of São Paulo, Ribeirão Preto, São Paulo, Brazil

References

[1] Mafong DD, Shin EJ, Lalwani AK: Use of laboratory evaluation and radiologic imaging in the diagnostic evaluation of children with sensorineural hearing loss. Laryngoscope. 2002;112:1-7.

[2] Baumgartner WD, Pok SM, Egelierler B, Franz P, Gstoettner W, Hamzavi J: The role of age in pediatric cochlear implantation. Int. J. Pediatr. Otorhinolaryngol. 2002;62(3): 223-228.

[3] Valencia DM, Rimell FL, Friedman BJ, Oblander MR, Helmbrecht J: Cochlear implantation in infants less than 12 months ages. Int. J. Pediatr. Otorhinolaryngol. 2008;72:767-773.

[4] Zwolan TA. Selection criteria and evaluation. In: S. Waltzman and N. Cohen, editors. *Cochlear implants*. New York: Theime; 2000. p. 63-73.

[5] Alpiner JG, McCarthy PA. Rehabilitative audiology: children and adults. 3rd. ed. Philadelphia: Lippincott Williams & Wilkings; 2000. 672p.

[6] Geers AE: Speech, language and reading skills after early cochlear implantation. Arch. Otolaryngol. Head Neck Surg. 2004;130(5):634-663.

[7] Nicholas JG, Geers AE: Will they catch up? The role of age at cochlear implantation in the spoken language development of children with severe to profound hearing loss. J. Speech Lang. Hear. Res. 2007;50(4):1048-1062.

[8] Litovsky RY, Godar SP: Experience with bilateral cochlear implants improves sound localization acuity in children. Otol. Neurotol. 2010;31(8):1287-1292.

[9] Mildner V, Sindija B, Zrinski KV: Speech perception of children with cochlear implants and children with traditional hearing aids. Clin. Linguist. Phon. 2006;20(2): 219-229.

[10] Osberger MJ: Clinical trial of the CLARION cochlear implant in children. Ann. Otol. Rhinol. Laryngol. 1999;177:88-92.

[11] Svirsky MA, Meyer TA: Comparison of speech perception in pediatric CLARION cochlear implant and hearing aid users. Ann. Otol. Rhinol. Laryngol. 1999;177:104-109.

[12] Tomblin JB: A comparison of language achievement in children with cochlear implants and children using hearing aids. J. Speech Lang. Hear. Res. 1999;42(2):497-511.

[13] Vanden BS: Assessment of basal sound identification skills and communication abilities in profoundly deaf children fitted with hearing aids or a cochlear implant. Clin. Otolaryngol. Allied Sci. 1998;23(5):455-461.

[14] Kuhn-Inacker H: Bilateral cochlear implants: a way to optimize auditory perception abilities in deaf children? Int. J. Pediatr. Otorhinolaryngol. 2004;68(10):1257-1266.

[15] Litovsky RY: Bilateral cochlear implants in children: localization acuity measured with minimum audible angle. Ear Hear. 2006;27(1):43-59.

[16] Peters BR: Importance of age and postimplantation experience on speech perception measures in children with sequential bilateral cochlear implants. Otol. Neurotol. 2007;29(5):649-657.

[17] Litovsky RY, Johnstone PM, Godar SP: Benefits of bilateral cochlear implants and/or hearing aids in children. Int. J. Audiol. 2006;45:S78-S91.

[18] Cyne JJ: Bilateral paediatric cochlear implants: a critical review. Int. J. Audiol. 2009;48:601-617.

[19] Brown KD, Balkany TJ: Benefits of bilateral cochlear implantation: a review. Curr. Opin. Otolaryngol. Head Neck Surg. 2007;15:315-318.

[20] Ching TY, Vanwanrooy E, Dillon H: Binaural-bimodal fitting or bilateral implantation for managing severe to profound deafness: a review. Trends Amplif. 2007;11:161-192.

[21] Murphy J, O'Donoghue G: Bilateral cochlear implantation: an evidence-based medicine evaluation. Laryngoscope. 2007;117:1412-1418.

[22] Schafer EC, Amlani AM, Seibold A, Shattuck PL: A metaanalytic comparison of binaural benefits between bilateral cochlear implants and bimodal stimulation. J. Am. Acad. Audiol. 2007;18:760-776.

[23] Tyler RS: Update on bilateral cochlear implantation. Curr. Opin. Otolaryngol. Head Neck Surg. 2003;11:388-393.

[24] Summerfield AQ: Selfreported benefits from successive bilateral cochlear implantation in post-lingually deafened adults: randomised controlled trial. Int. J. Audiol. 2006;45(1):S99-S107.

[25] Peters BR: Importance of age and postimplantation experience on speech perception measures in children with sequential bilateral cochlear implants. Otol. Neurotol. 2007;29(5):649-657.

[26] Litovsky RY, Parkinson A, Arcaroli J: Bilateral cochlear implants in adults and children. Arch. Otolaryngol. Head Neck Surg. 2004;130:648-655.

[27] Grantham DW, Ashmead DH, Ricketts TA: Horizontal-plane localization of noise and speech signals by postlingually deafened adults fitted with bilateral cochlear implants. Ear Hear. 2007;28:524-541.

[28] Neuman AC, Haravon A, Sislian N: Sound direction identification with bilateral cochlear implants. Ear Hear. 2007;28:73-82.

[29] Schafer EC, Amlani AM, Seibold A, Shattuck PL: A meta-analytic comparison of binaural benefits between bilateral cochlear implants and bimodal stimulation. J. Am. Acad. Audiol. 2007;18(9):760-776.

[30] Wie OB: Language development in children after receiving bilateral cochlear implants between 5 and 18 months. Int. J. Otorhinolaryngol. 2010;74(11):1258-1266.

[31] Bauer PW, Sharma A, Dorman M: Central auditory development in children with bilateral cochlear implants. Arch. Otolaryngol. Head Neck Surg. 2006;1132(10): 1133-1136.

[32] Gordon KA, Valero J, Papsin BC: Binaural processing in children using bilateral cochlear implants. Neuroreport. 2007;18(6):613-617.

[33] Mok M, Hughes KC, Galvin KL: Can adolescents and Young adults with prelingual hearing loss benefit from a second, sequential cochlear implant. Int. J. Audio. 2010;49(5):368-377.

[34] Papsin BC, Gordon KA: Bilateral cochlear implants should be the standard for children with bilateral sensorineural deafness. Otolaryngol. Head Neck Surg. 2008;16:69-74.